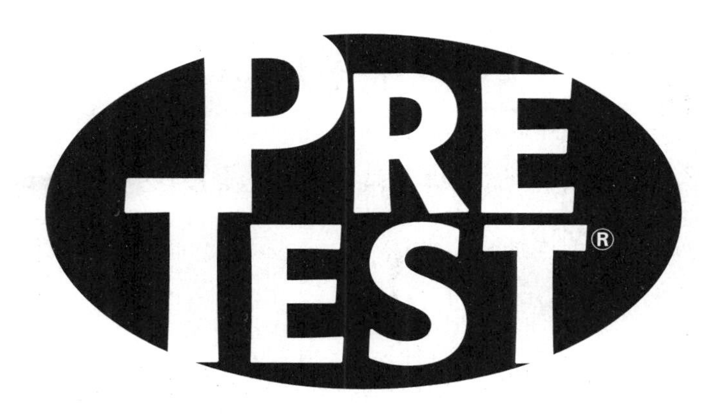

Medicine

PreTest® Self-Assessment and Review

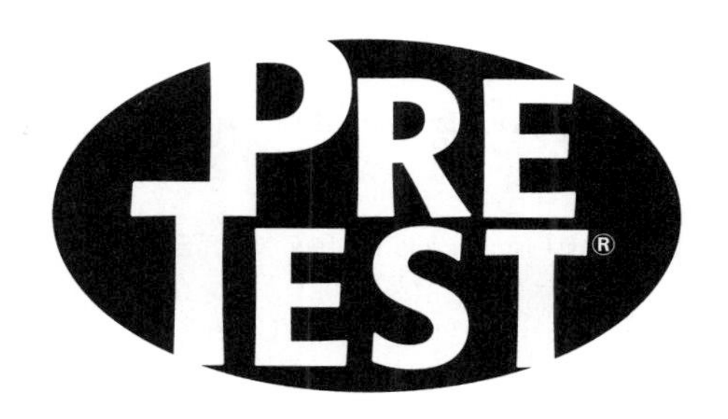

Medicine

PreTest® Self-Assessment and Review

Ninth Edition

STEVEN L. BERK, M.D.

Regional Dean
Professor of Medicine
Texas Tech University School of Medicine at Amarillo
Amarillo, Texas

WILLIAM R. DAVIS, M.D.

Chairman and Associate Professor
Department of Internal Medicine
Texas Tech University School of Medicine at Amarillo
Amarillo, Texas

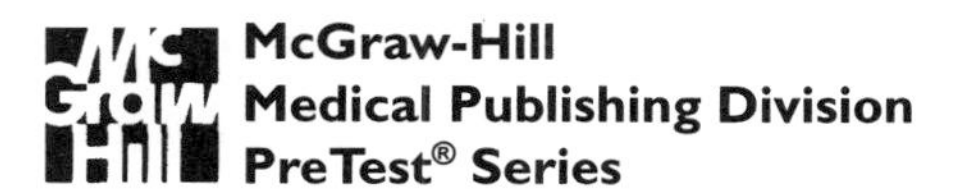

McGraw-Hill
Medical Publishing Division
PreTest® Series

NEW YORK ST. LOUIS SAN FRANCISCO AUCKLAND
BOGOTÁ CARACAS LISBON LONDON MADRID
MEXICO CITY MILAN MONTREAL NEW DELHI
SAN JUAN SINGAPORE SYDNEY TOKYO TORONTO

McGraw-Hill

*A Division of The **McGraw-Hill** Companies*

Medicine: PreTest® Self-Assessment and Review, Ninth Edition

1 2 3 4 5 6 7 8 9 0 DOC/DOC 0 9 8 7 6 5 4 3 2 1 0

ISBN 0-07-135960-5

This book was set in Berkeley by North Market Street Graphics.
The editor was Catherine A. Wenz.
The production supervisor was Rohnda Barnes.
Project management was provided by North Market Street Graphics.
The text designer was Jim Sullivan / RepCat Graphics & Editorial Services.
The cover designer was Li Chen Chang / Pinpoint.
R.R. Donnelley & Sons was printer and binder.

This book is printed on acid-free paper.

Library of Congress Cataloging-in-Publication Data

Medicine : PreTest self-assessment and review.—9th ed. / editors, Steven L. Berk, William R. Davis.
p. ; cm.
At head of title: PreTest
Includes bibliographical references.
ISBN 0-07-135960-5
1. Medicine—Examinations, questions, etc. I. Berk, S. L. (Steven L.), 1949– II. Davis, William R., 1951–
[DNLM: 1. Medicine—Examination Questions. W 18.2 M4914 2000]
R834.5 .M4 2000
616'.0076—dc21 00-030562

This book is printed on acid-free paper.

Hematology and Oncology

Neurology

Dermatology

General Medicine and Prevention

Allergy and Immunology

Introduction

Medicine: PreTest® Self-Assessment and Review, Ninth Edition, is intended to provide medical students, as well as house officers and physicians, with a convenient tool for assessing and improving their knowledge of medicine. The 500 questions in this book are similar in format and complexity to those included in Step 2 of the United States Medical Licensing Examination (USMLE). They may also be a useful study tool for Step 3.

Each question in this book has a corresponding answer, a reference to a text that provides background for the answer, and a short discussion of various issues raised by the question and its answer. A listing of references for the entire book follows the last chapter.

To simulate the time constraints imposed by the qualifying examinations for which this book is intended as a practice guide, the student or physician should allot about one minute for each question. After answering all questions in a chapter, as much time as necessary should be spent reviewing the explanations for each question at the end of the chapter. Attention should be given to all explanations, even if the examinee answered the question correctly. Those seeking more information on a subject should refer to the reference materials listed or to other standard texts in medicine.

ACKNOWLEDGMENTS

We would like to offer special thanks to

Our wives, Shirley Berk and Janet Davis, for moral support and helpful suggestions concerning the format of the questions

Our children, Jeremy Berk, Justin Berk, Abby Davis, and Kyle Davis, for their computer expertise

Our staff, Margie McAlister, Jackie Hammett, and Donna Forrester, for excellent support in organizing, collating, and typing the manuscript

To Texas Tech University School of Medicine at Amarillo—in the pursuit of excellence

To students of Texas Tech University School of Medicine, for review of the text.

The publisher wishes to thank Carol Bunten, a medical student from the University of Iowa College of Medicine, for reviewing this manuscript prior to publication.

INFECTIOUS DISEASE

DIRECTIONS: Each item below contains a question or incomplete statement followed by suggested responses. Select the **one best** response to each question.

1. A 30-year-old male patient has complained of fever and sore throat for several days. The patient presents to you today with additional complaints of hoarseness, difficulty breathing, and drooling. On examination, the patient is febrile and has inspiratory wheezes. Which of the following would be the best course of action?

a. Begin outpatient treatment with ampicillin
b. Culture throat for beta-hemolytic streptococci
c. Admit to intensive care unit and obtain otolaryngology consultation
d. Schedule for chest x-ray

2. A 70-year-old patient with longstanding type 2 diabetes mellitus presents with complaints of pain in the left ear with purulent drainage. On physical exam, the patient is afebrile. The pinna of the left ear is tender, and the external auditory canal is swollen and edematous. The peripheral white blood cell count is normal. The organism most likely to grow from the purulent drainage is

a. *Pseudomonas aeruginosa*
b. *Staphylococcus aureus*
c. *Candida albicans*
d. *Haemophilus influenzae*
e. *Moraxella catarrhalis*

Items 3–4

A 25-year-old male student presents with a chief complaint of rash. There is no headache, fever, or myalgia. A slightly pruritic maculopapular rash is noted over the abdomen, trunk, palms of hands, and soles of feet. Inguinal, occipital, and cervical lymphadenopathy is also noted. Hypertrophic, flat, wartlike lesions are noted around the anal area. Laboratory studies show the following:

Hct: 40%
Hgb: 14 g/dL
WBC: 13,000/mm^3
Diff
Segmented neutrophils: 50%
Lymphocytes: 50%

3. The most useful laboratory test in this patient is

a. Weil-Felix titer
b. Venereal Disease Research Laboratory (VDRL) test
c. *Chlamydia* titer
d. Blood cultures

4. The treatment of choice for this patient would be

a. Penicillin
b. Ceftriaxone
c. Tetracycline
d. Interferon alpha
e. Erythromycin

Items 5–7

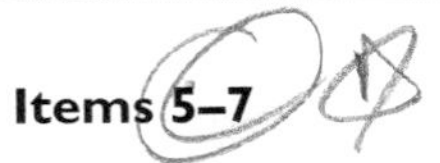

A 20-year-old female college student presents with a five-day history of cough, low-grade fever (temperature 100°F), sore throat, and coryza. On exam, there is mild conjunctivitis and pharyngitis. Tympanic membranes are inflamed and one bullous lesion is seen. Chest exam shows few basilar rales. Laboratory findings are as follows:

Hct: 38
WBC: 12,000/mm^3
Lymphocytes: 50%
Mean corpuscular volume (MCV): 83 μm^3
Reticulocytes: 3% of red cells
CXR: Bilateral patchy lower lobe infiltrates

5. The sputum Gram stain is likely to show

a. Gram-positive diplococci
b. Tiny gram-negative coccobacilli
c. White blood cells without organisms
d. Tubercle bacilli

6. This patient is likely to have

a. High titers of adenovirus
b. High titers of IgM cold agglutinins
c. A positive silver methenamine stain
d. A positive blood culture for *Streptococcus pneumoniae*

7. Treatment of choice would be

a. Erythromycin
b. Supportive therapy
c. Trimethoprim-sulfamethoxazole
d. Cefuroxime

Items 8–10

A 19-year-old male presents with a one-week history of malaise and anorexia followed by fever and sore throat. On physical examination, the throat is inflamed without exudate. There are a few palatal petechiae. Cervical adenopathy is present. The liver is percussed at 12 cm and the spleen is palpable.

Throat culture: negative for group A streptococci
Hct: 38%
Hgb: 12 g/dL
Reticulocytes: 4%
WBC: 14,000 mm^3
Segmented: 30%
Lymphocytes: 60%
Monocytes: 10%
Bilirubin total: 2.0 mg/dL (n 0.2 to 1.2)
Lactic dehydrogenase (LDH) serum: 260 IU/L (n 20 to 220)
Aspartate (AST): 40 U/L (n 8 to 20 U/L)
Alanine (ALT): 35 U/L (n 8 to 20 U/L)
Alkaline phosphatase: 40 IU/L (n 35 to 125)

8. The most important initial test would be

a. Liver biopsy
b. Strep screen
c. Peripheral blood smear
d. Toxoplasmosis IgG
e. Lymph node biopsy

9. The most important serum test is

a. Heterophile antibody
b. Hepatitis B IgM
c. Cytomegalovirus IgG
d. ASLO titer
e. Hepatitis C antibody

10. Corticosteroids would be indicated if

a. Liver function tests worsen
b. Fatigue lasts more than one week
c. Severe hemolytic anemia is demonstrated
d. Hepatitis B is confirmed

DIRECTIONS: Each group of questions below consists of lettered headings followed by a set of numbered items. For each numbered item, select the **one** lettered heading with which it is most closely associated. Each lettered heading may be used once, more than once, or not at all.

Items 11–14

Match the clinical description with the most likely organism.

a. *Streptococcus pneumoniae*
b. *Staphylococcus aureus*
c. *Viridans streptococci*
d. *Providencia stuartii*
e. *Actinomyces israelii*
f. *Haemophilus ducreyi*
g. *Neisseria meningitidis*
h. *Listeria monocytogenes*

11. A 30-year-old female with mitral valve prolapse and mitral regurgitant murmur develops fever, weight loss, and anorexia after undergoing dental procedure.

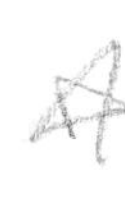

12. An 80-year-old-male, hospitalized for hip fracture, has Foley catheter in place when he develops shaking chill, fever, and hypotension.

13. A young man develops painless, fluctuant, purplish lesion over the mandible. Cutaneous fistula is noted after several weeks.

14. A sickle cell anemia patient presents with high fever, toxicity, signs of pneumonia, and stiff neck.

Items 15–18.

Select one antiviral agent for each patient.

a. Ganciclovir
b. Acyclovir
c. Interferon alpha
d. Didanosine
e. Ribavirin
f. Amantadine
g. Vidarabine
h. Zalcitabine

15. Military recruit develops pneumonia secondary to influenza A. Symptoms began 24 hours prior to physician visit.

16. HIV-positive patient with CD4 count of 50 complains of onset visual blurring; opacity seen on fundoscopic exam.

17. Sexually active young woman has anogenital warts, requests intralesional therapy.

18. Infant with respiratory syncytial virus infection requires mechanical ventilation.

Items 19–21

Match the fungal agent most likely responsible for the disease process described below.

a. *Histoplasma capsulatum*
b. *Blastomycosis dermatitidis*
c. *Coccidioides immitis*
d. *Cryptococcus neoformans*
e. *Candida albicans*
f. *Aspergillus fumigatus*
g. *Zygomycosis*

19. Fever, cough, and weight loss in young, previously healthy male. Presents with verrucous skin lesions and bone pain. Chest x-ray shows nodular infiltrates.

20. Diabetic patient is admitted with elevated blood sugar and acidosis. Complains of headache and sinus tenderness. Has black, necrotic material draining from nares.

21. Young woman with asthma, eosinophilia. Fleeting pulmonary infiltrates occur with bronchial plugging.

DIRECTIONS: Each item below contains a question or incomplete statement followed by suggested responses. Select the **one best** response to each question.

Items 22–24

A 40-year-old male develops bilateral facial weakness. The patient returned from a camping trip in Wisconsin that had lasted six weeks. The patient gives a history of arthralgias. On exam, he cannot close either eye well or raise either eyebrow. The first heart sound is diminished. There is no evidence of arthritis.

Hgb: 14 g/dL
WBC: 10,000/mm^3
VDRL: Negative
FTA-Abs: Positive
EKG: First-degree AV block

22. Which of the following would be most useful?

a. CT scan of head
b. MRI of head
c. More detailed history
d. Kveim test

23. The likely cause of these symptoms is

a. Intracranial infection
b. Lyme disease
c. Endocarditis
d. Herpes simplex

24. Treatment of choice would be

a. Penicillin or ceftriaxone
b. Acyclovir
c. Corticosteroids
d. Aminoglycoside

25. You are a physician in charge of the patients that reside in a nursing home. Several of the patients have developed influenza-like symptoms, and the community is in the midst of an influenza A outbreak. None of the nursing home residents have received the influenza vaccine. What course of action would be most appropriate?

a. Give the influenza vaccine to all residents of the nursing home who do not have a contraindication to the vaccine (allergy to eggs)
b. Give the influenza vaccine to all residents of the nursing home who do not have a contraindication to the vaccine. Also give amantadine for a two-week period
c. Give amantadine alone to all nursing home residents
d. Do not give any prophylactic regimen

26. Which of the following statements concerning cryptococcal meningoencephalitis is correct?

a. It may occur in patients with no identifiable immunological defect
b. Urine and blood cultures are always negative
c. The india ink preparation usually reveals gram-negative bacteria
d. Detection of cryptococcal polysaccharide antigen in cerebrospinal fluid (CSF) is sensitive but nonspecific

27. Patients with cellular immune dysfunction are least susceptible to infection with which of the following organisms?

a. Cytomegalovirus
b. *Haemophilus influenzae*
c. *Mycobacterium tuberculosis*
d. *Pneumocystis carinii*
e. *Histoplasma capsulatum*

28. A 30-year-old man who has spent 5 of the last 10 years in prison in New York City is referred from the prison because of hemoptysis. He has a history of tuberculosis diagnosed three years ago and took isoniazid and rifampin for about a month. A cavitary lesion is seen on chest x-ray. One should do all the following *except*

a. Obtain sputum for acid-fast bacilli (AFB) stain, culture, and sensitivity
b. Start supervised isoniazid and rifampin administration
c. Start a supervised multiple drug combination to treat multidrug-resistant tuberculosis
d. Place the patient in respiratory isolation
e. Perform routine screening of inmates and staff for tuberculosis

29. A recent outbreak of severe diarrhea is currently being investigated. Several children developed bloody diarrhea, and one remains hospitalized with acute renal failure. A preliminary investigation has determined that all the affected children ate at the same restaurant. The food they consumed was most likely to be

a. Pork chops
b. Hamburger
c. Gefilte fish
d. Sushi
e. Soft-boiled eggs

30. A 40-year-old female nurse was admitted to the hospital because of fever to 103°F. Despite a thorough workup in the hospital for over three weeks, no etiology has been found, and she continues to have temperature spikes greater than 102°F. The least likely diagnosis in this patient

a. Occult bacterial infection
b. Influenza
c. Lymphoma
d. Adult Still's disease
e. Factitious fever

31. In a patient who has mitral valve insufficiency, which procedure does not require prophylactic antibiotic therapy?

a. Cardiac catheterization
b. Prostatectomy
c. Cystoscopy
d. Tonsillectomy
e. Periodontal surgery

32. Rabies, an acute viral disease of the mammalian central nervous system, is transmitted by infective secretions, usually saliva. Which of the following statements about this disease is correct?

a. The disease is caused by a reovirus that elicits both complement-fixing and hemagglutinating antibodies useful in the diagnosis of the disease
b. The incubation period is variable, and, although 10 days is the most common elapsed time between infection and symptoms, some cases remain asymptomatic for 30 days
c. Only 30% of infected patients will survive
d. In the United States, the skunk and the raccoon have been important recent sources of human disease
e. Wild animals that have bitten and are suspected of being rabid should be killed and their brains examined for virus particles by electron microscopy

DIRECTIONS: Each group of questions below consists of lettered headings followed by a set of numbered items. For each numbered item select the **one** lettered heading with which it is most closely associated. Each lettered heading may be used once, more than once, or not at all.

Items 33–36

Match each clinical description with the appropriate infectious agent.

a. Herpes simplex virus
b. Epstein-Barr virus
c. Parvovirus B19
d. *Staphylococcus aureus*
e. *Neisseria meningitidis*

33. "Slapped-cheek" rash

34. Desquamation of skin on hands and feet

35. Petechiae on trunk

36. Diffuse rash after administration of ampicillin

Items 37–41

Match the following diseases with their appropriate signs.

a. Koplik's spots
b. Agammaglobulinemia
c. A vesicular and pustular eruption that begins when the patient is afebrile
d. Acute cerebellar ataxia
e. Pancreatitis

37. Mumps

38. Chickenpox

39. Smallpox

40. Echovirus infection

41. Measles

Items 42–46

Match the clinical illness with the appropriate opportunistic pathogen in patients with AIDS.

a. *Pneumocystis carinii*
b. *Toxoplasma gondii*
c. *Cryptosporidium*
d. Cytomegalovirus
e. *Salmonella*

42. Pneumonia

43. Retinitis

44. Seizures

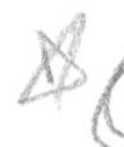

45. Bacteremia

46. Diarrhea diagnosed by direct examination of stool

Items 47–51

For each of the sexually transmitted diseases listed below, select the treatment of choice.

a. Penicillin
b. Doxycycline
c. Ceftriaxone plus doxycycline
d. Metronidazole
e. Acyclovir

47. Presumed gonococcal urethritis

48. Nongonococcal urethritis

49. Severe primary genital herpes

50. Trichomoniasis

51. Syphilis

Items 52–55

Identify the antimicrobial agent associated with the adverse effects listed below.

a. Gentamicin
b. Imipenem
c. Tetracycline
d. Clindamycin

52. Photosensitivity

53. Acute tubular necrosis

54. Progressive weakness in a patient with myasthenia gravis

55. Seizures

DIRECTIONS: Each item below contains a question or incomplete statement followed by suggested responses. Select the **one best** response to each question.

56. A previously healthy 25-year-old music teacher develops fever and a rash over her face and chest. The rash is itchy and on exam involves multiple papules and vesicles in varying stages of development. One week later she complains of cough and is found to have an infiltrate on x-ray. The most likely etiology of the infection is

a. *Streptococcus pneumoniae*
b. *Mycoplasma pneumoniae*
c. *Pneumocystis carinii*
d. Varicella virus

Items 57–58

57. A 22-year-old male complains of fever and shortness of breath. There is no pleuritic chest pain or rigors, and there is no sputum production. A chest x-ray shows diffuse perihilar infiltrates. The patient worsens while on erythromycin. A silver methenamine stain shows cystlike structures. Which of the following is correct?

a. Definitive diagnosis can be made by serology
b. The organism will grow after 48 hours
c. History will likely provide important clues to the diagnosis
d. Cavitary disease is likely to develop

58. Which of the following statements about the treatment of the above patient is correct?

a. Oral antibiotic therapy is never appropriate
b. Trimethoprim-sulfamethoxazole is the treatment of choice in the nonallergic patient
c. Concomitant corticosteroids should always be avoided
d. Tetracycline is more effective than erythromycin

59. A 25-year-old male from East Tennessee had been ill for five days with fever, chills, and headache when he noted a rash that developed on his palms and soles. In addition to macular lesions, petechiae are noted on the wrists and ankles. The patient has spent the summer camping. The most important fact to be determined in the history is

a. Exposure to contaminated springwater
b. Exposure to raw pork
c. Exposure to ticks
d. Exposure to prostitutes

60. A 19-year-old male has a history of athlete's foot but is otherwise healthy when he develops the sudden onset of fever and pain in the right foot and leg. On physical exam, the foot and leg are fiery red with a well-defined indurated margin that appears to be rapidly advancing. There is tender inguinal lymphadenopathy. The most likely organism to cause this infection is

a. *Staphylococcus epidermidis*
b. Tinea pedis
c. *Streptococcus pyogenes*
d. Mixed anerobic infection

61. An 18-year-old male has been seen in clinic for urethral discharge. He is treated with ceftriaxone but the discharge has not resolved and the culture has returned as no growth. The most likely etiologic agent to cause this infection is

a. Ceftriaxone-resistant gonococci
b. *Chlamydia psittaci*
c. *Chlamydia trachomatis*
d. Herpes simplex

DIRECTIONS: Each group of questions below consists of lettered headings followed by a set of numbered items. For each numbered item select the **one** lettered heading with which it is most closely associated. Each lettered heading may be used once, more than once, or not at all.

Items 62–68

Match the clinical description with the most likely etiologic agent.

a. *Candida albicans*
b. *Aspergillus flavus*
c. *Coccidioides immitis*
d. Herpes simplex—type 1
e. Herpes simpex virus—type 2
f. Hantavirus
g. *Tropheryma whippelii*
h. Coxsackievirus B
i. *Histopasmosis capsultatum*
j. Human parvovirus
k. *Cryptococcus neoformans*

62. HIV-positive patient develops fever and dysphagia; endoscopic biopsy shows yeast and hyphae.

63. A 50-year-old develops sudden onset of bizarre behavior. CSF shows 80 lymphocytes; magnetic resonance imaging has temporal lobe abnormalities.

64. Previous history of tuberculosis; patient now complains of hemoptysis. Has upper lobe mass with cavity, crescent-shaped air-fluid level.

65. Filipino patient develops pulmonary nodule after travel through Southwest.

66. A 35-year-old male had fever, cough, sore throat. After several days develops chest pain with diffuse ST segment elevations on EKG.

67. Overwhelming pneumonia with adult respiratory distress syndrome occurs on Indian reservation in Southwest following exposure to deer mouse.

68. Child develops erythematous rash, appearing as "slapped cheek."

INFECTIOUS DISEASE

Answers

1. The answer is c. *(Gorbach, 2/e, pp 542–544.)* This patient, with the development of hoarseness, breathing difficulty, and stridor, is likely to have developed acute epiglottitis. Because of the possibility of impending airway obstruction, the patient should be admitted to an intensive care unit for close monitoring. The diagnosis can be confirmed by indirect laryngoscopy or soft tissue x-rays of the neck, which may show an enlarged epiglottis. Otolaryngology consult should be obtained. The most likely organism causing this infection is *H. influenzae*. Many of these organisms are beta lactamase–producing and would be resistant to ampicillin. The clinical findings are not consistent with the presentation of streptococcal pharyngitis. Lateral neck film would be more useful than chest x-ray.

2. The answer is a. *(Harrison, 13/e, p 518.)* Ear pain and drainage in an elderly diabetic patient must raise concern about malignant external otitis. The swelling and inflammation of the external auditory meatus strongly suggests this diagnosis. This infection usually occurs in older diabetics and is almost always caused by *P. aeruginosa*. *H. influenzae* and *M. catarrhalis* frequently cause otitis media, but not external otitis.

3–4. The answers are 3-b, 4-a. *(Fauci, 14/e, pp 1026–1027.)* The diffuse rash involving palms and soles would in itself suggest the possibility of secondary syphilis. The hypertrophic, wartlike lesions around the anal area are called *condyloma lata,* which are specific for secondary syphilis. The VDRL slide test will be positive in all patients with secondary syphilis. The Weil-Felix titer has been used as a screening test for rickettsial infection. In this patient, who has condyloma and no systemic symptoms, Rocky Mountain spotted fever would be unlikely. No chlamydial infection would present in this way. Blood cultures might be drawn to rule out bacterial infection such as chronic meningococcemia; however, the clinical picture is not consistent with a systemic bacterial infection. Penicillin is the drug of choice for secondary syphilis. Ceftriaxone and tetracycline are usually considered to be alternative therapies. Interferon alpha has been used in the treatment of condyloma acuminata, a lesion that can be mistaken for syphilitic condyloma.

5–7. The answers are 5-c, 6-b, 7-a. *(Fauci, 14/e, pp 1053–1054.)* This young woman presents with symptoms of both upper and lower respiratory infection. The combination of sore throat, bullous myringitis, and infiltrates on chest x-ray is consistent with infection due to *M. pneumoniae.* This minute organism is not seen on Gram stain. Neither *S. pneumoniae* nor *H. influenzae* would produce this combination of upper and lower respiratory tract symptoms. The patient is likely to have high titers of IgM cold agglutinins. The low hematocrit and elevated reticulocyte count reflect a hemolytic anemia which can occur from mycoplasma infection. These IgM-class antibodies are directed to the I antigen on the erythrocyte membrane. The treatment of choice for mycoplasma infection is erythromycin.

8–10. The answers are 8-c, 9-a, 10-c. *(Fauci, 14/e, pp 1089–1090.)* This young man presents with classic signs and symptoms of infectious mononucleosis. In a young patient with fever, pharyngitis, lymphadenopathy, and lymphocytosis, the peripheral blood smear should be evaluated for atypical lymphocytes. A heterophile antibody test should be performed. The symptoms described in association with atypical lymphocytes and a positive heterophile test are virtually always due to Epstein-Barr virus. Neither liver biopsy nor lymph node biopsy are necessary. Workup for toxoplasmosis or cytomegalovirus infection, hepatitis B and C would be considered in heterophile-negative patients, Hepatitis does not occur in the setting of rheumatic fever, and an antistreptolysin O titer is not indicated. Corticosteroids are indicated in the treatment of infectious mononucleosis when severe hemolytic anemia is demonstrated or when airway obstruction occurs. Neither fatigue nor the complication of hepatitis are indications for corticosteroid therapy.

11–14. The answers are 11-c, 12-d, 13-e, 14-a. *(Fauci, 14/e, pp 785–787, 871, 989, 936.)* This 30-year-old-female with mitral valve prolapse has developed subacute bacterial endocarditis. The likely etiologic agent is a *Viridans streptococci. Viridans streptococci* cause most cases of subacute bacterial endocarditis. No other agent listed is likely to cause this infection. The 80-year-old-male with a Foley catheter in place has developed a nosocomial infection likely secondary to urosepsis. *Providencia* species frequently cause urinary tract infection in the hospitalized patient. The young man with a fluctuant lesion and fistula over the mandible presents a classic picture of cervicofacial actinomycosis. The sickle cell anemia patient who presents with concomitant pneumonia and meningitis has overwhelming infection with *S. pneumoniae. S. pneumoniae* is a particularly severe infection associated with sickle cell disease.

15–18. The answers are 15-f, 16-a, 17-c, 18-e. *(Fauci, 14/e, pp 1072–1079.)* Amantadine has been shown to alter the course of influenza A favorably, particularly when begun within 48 hours of the start of symptoms. The HIV-positive patient with a low CD4 count and visual blurring has developed cytomegalovirus retinitis. Gancyclovir is the drug of choice (foscarnet has also been used effectively). Interferon alpha has been approved for intralesional therapy of condyloma acuminatum, venereal warts caused by papilloma virus. Ribavirin improves mortality in mechanically ventilated infants with RSV infection.

19–21. The answers are 19-b, 20-g, 21-e. *(Fauci, 14/e, pp 1148–1158.)* Blastomycosis presents with signs and symptoms of chronic respiratory infection. The organism has a tendency to produce skin lesions in exposed areas that become crusted, ulcerated, or verrucous. Bone pain is caused by osteolytic lesions. Mucormycosis is a zygomycosis that originates in the nose and paranasal sinuses. Sinus tenderness, bloody nasal discharge, and obtundation occur usually in the setting of diabetic ketoacidosis. Aspergillus can result in several different infectious processes, including aspergilloma, disseminated aspergillus in the immunocompromised patient, or allergic bronchopulmonary aspergillosis. Bronchopulmonary aspergillosis is the most likely diagnosis in this young woman with asthma and eosinophilia. Bronchial plugs, often filled with hyphal forms, result in repeated infiltrates and exacerbation of wheezing.

22–24. The answers are 22-c, 23-b, 24-a. *(Fauci, 14/e, pp 1042–1044.)* This patient presents with a symptom complex that includes facial nerve palsies, arthralgia, and first-degree AV block. Facial nerve palsy has been increasingly recognized as a first manifestation of Lyme disease. Within several weeks of the onset of illness, about 8% of patients develop cardiac involvement, with heart block being the most common manifestation. During this stage of early disseminated infection, musculoskeletal pain is common. The diagnosis of Lyme disease is based on careful history and physical exam with serologic confirmation by detection of antibody to *Borrelia burgdorferi*. Neither CT or MRI of head would be indicated, as lesion is a peripheral facial palsy. Sarcoidosis can also cause both facial nerve palsy and AV block but it is much less likely, and the Kveim test is rarely used to pursue this diagnosis. The treatment of choice for Lyme disease at this stage would be penicillin or ceftriaxone.

25. The answer is b. *(Fauci, 14/e, pp 1115–1116.)* Influenza A is a potentially lethal disease in the elderly and chronically debilitated patient. In institutional settings such as nursing homes, outbreaks are likely to be particularly severe. Hence, prophylaxis is extremely important in this setting. All residents should receive the vaccine unless they have known egg allergy (patients can choose to decline the vaccine). Since protective antibody to the vaccine will not develop for two weeks, amantadine can be used for protection against Influenza A during the interim two-week period. A reduced dose is given to elderly patients.

26. The answer is a. *(Stobo, 23/e, pp 555–556.)* Meningitis or meningoencephalitis is the most common clinical manifestation of infection with the fungus *C. neoformans*. The majority of patients are immunocompromised (i.e., they are receiving corticosteroid or immunosuppressive therapy or are infected with HIV), but about 35% have no identifiable predisposing immunological defect. The diagnosis is confirmed by examination of the CSF. The India ink preparation of CSF will reveal budding yeast in about three-fourths of cases. Cryptococcal polysaccharide antigen is present in CSF in over 90% of cases; in most cases this antigen is also present in serum and is highly specific. Culture of CSF is usually positive; cultures of blood and urine are each positive for cryptococci in about one-fourth of patients.

27. The answer is b. *(Mandell, 4/e, pp 149–156.)* Patients with Hodgkin's disease or AIDS or those receiving corticosteroid and cytotoxic agents all have in common a dysfunction of cellular immunity that leaves them particularly susceptible to infection with such pathogens as *L. monocytogenes, Legionella, Nocardia, Salmonella*, varicella-zoster virus, herpes simplex virus, *T. gondii*, and *Strongyloides stercoralis*, as well as those listed in the question. Patients with humoral immune dysfunction, in contrast, lack opsonizing antibodies in their serum and therefore cannot adequately defend against encapsulated organisms such as *H. influenzae* and *S. pneumoniae.* Granulocytopenic patients and those with defective leukocyte phagocytic activity are prone to infection with *Candida, Aspergillus,* agents of mucormycosis, *P. aeruginosa,* and certain other bacteria.

28. The answer is b. *(CDC, MMWR 42:48–51, 1993.)* Multidrug-resistant tuberculosis (TB) has become an increasing problem in several settings, including correctional facilities and health care institutions. Noncompliance or poor compliance with prescribed anti-TB medications is the major factor in the development of multiple drug resistance. When the disease is suspected, patients should be placed in respiratory isolation and sputum should be obtained for AFB stain, culture, and sensitivity. Treatment of high-risk patients, such as this patient, should be supervised and the possibility of multidrug resistance should be considered. Regular screening of inmates and staff for TB is important for preventing the spread of TB within the facility and for early diagnosis of new infections.

29. The answer is b. *(CDC, MMWR 42:258–263, 1993.)* The outbreak described is similar to those previously attributed to *Escherichia coli* 0157:H7. Ingestion and infection with this organism may result in a spectrum of illnesses, including mild diarrhea, hemorrhagic colitis with bloody diarrhea, acute renal failure, and death. Infection has been associated with ingestion of contaminated beef, in particular ground beef, but also raw milk and contamination via the fecal-oral route. Cooking ground beef so that it is no longer pink is an effective means of preventing infection, as are hand washing and pasteurization of milk.

30. The answer is b. *(Stobo, 23/e, pp 547–551.)* Patients may develop fever as a result of infectious and noninfectious diseases. The term *fever of unknown origin* (FUO) is applied when significant fever persists without a known cause after an adequate evaluation. Several studies have found the leading causes of FUO to include infections, malignancies, collagen vascular diseases, and granulomatous diseases. As the ability to more rapidly diagnose some of these diseases increases, their likelihood of causing undiagnosed persistent fever lessens. Infections such as intraabdominal abscesses, tuberculosis, hepatobiliary disease, endocarditis (especially if the patient had previously taken antibiotics), and osteomyelitis may cause

FUO. In immunocompromised patients, such as those infected with HIV, a number of opportunistic infections or lymphoma may cause fever and escape early diagnosis. Self-limited infections such as influenza should not cause persistent fever for many weeks. Neoplastic diseases such as lymphomas and some solid tumors (e.g., hypernephroma and primary or metastatic disease of the liver) are associated with FUO. A number of collagen vascular diseases may cause FUO. Since conditions such as systemic lupus erythematosus are more easily diagnosed today, they are less frequent causes of this syndrome. Adult Still's disease, however, is often difficult to diagnose. Other causes of FUO include granulomatous diseases (which include giant cell arteritis, regional enteritis, sarcoidosis, and granulomatous hepatitis), drug fever, and peripheral pulmonary emboli. Factitious fever is most common among young adults employed in health-related positions. A prior psychiatric history or multiple hospitalizations at other institutions may be clues to this condition. Such patients may induce infections by self-injection of nonsterile material, with resultant multiple abscesses or polymicrobial infections. Alternatively, some patients may manipulate their thermometers. In these cases, a discrepancy between temperature and pulse or between oral temperature and witnessed rectal temperature will be observed.

31. The answer is a. *(Mandell, 4/e pp 793–798.)* Although no evidence exists that prophylactic antibiotic therapy prevents endocarditis, prophylaxis is recommended for all procedures that may generate bacteremias. Following cardiac catheterization, blood cultures obtained from a distal vein are rarely positive. Thus, prophylactic antibiotics are not currently recommended for cardiac catheterization. Bacteremia commonly occurs following other procedures such as periodontal surgery, tonsillectomy, and prostate surgery.

32. The answer is d. *(Mandell, 4/e, pp 1527–1540.)* Rabies is caused by a bullet-shaped rhabdovirus. In the United States, dogs are seldom rabid. The animals that represent the most danger are wild skunks and bats; foxes are also possible carriers. Raccoons are responsible for an increasing number of cases in the mid-Atlantic states. The incubation period ranges from 4 days to many years, but is usually between 20 and 90 days. The incubation period is usually shorter with a bite to the head than with one to an extremity. In humans, only three definite recoveries from established infection have been reported. Nonimmunized animals that have bitten should be killed and their brains submitted for virus immunofluorescent antibody examination. A negative fluorescent test removes the need to treat the bite victim, either actively or passively.

33–36. The answers are 33-c, 34-d, 35-e, 36-b. *(Gorbach, 2/e, pp 1334–1335, 1648, 1692, 1387.)* Parvovirus B19 is the agent responsible for erythema infectiosum, also known as *fifth disease.* This most commonly affects children between ages 5 and 14, but it can also occur in adults. The disease is characterized by a slapped-cheek rash, which may follow a prodrome of low-grade fever. A lacelike, diffuse rash may also occur. Complications in adults include arthralgias, arthritis, aplastic crisis in patients with chronic hemolytic anemia, spontaneous abortion, and hydrops fetalis.

Desquamation of the skin usually occurs during or after recovery from toxic shock syndrome (associated with a toxin produced by *S. aureus*). Peeling of the skin is also seen in Kawasaki disease, scarlet fever, and some severe drug reactions.

Petechial rashes are often seen with potentially life-threatening infections, including meningococcemia, gonococcemia, rickettsial disease, infective endocarditis, atypical measles, and disseminated intravascular coagulation (DIC) associated with sepsis.

Infectious mononucleosis is the usual manifestation of infection with Epstein-Barr virus. Since it is a viral disease, antibiotic therapy is not indicated. A diffuse maculopapular rash has been observed in over 90% of patients with infectious mononucleosis who are given ampicillin.

37–41. The answers are 37-e, 38-d, 39-c, 40-b, 41-a. *(Mandell, 4/e, pp 1345–1351, 1496–1501, 1519–1526.)* Although salivary adenitis is the most prominent feature of the communicable disease of viral-origin mumps, it is not uncommon to have involvement of the gonads, meninges, and pancreas. Males who develop mumps after the age of puberty have a 20 to 35% chance of developing a painful orchitis. Central nervous system involvement is common but usually mild, with 50% of cases having an increase in lymphocytes detectable in the CSF. Myocarditis, thrombocytopenic purpura, and polyarthritis may also occur as complications of this disease. An inflammatory change in the pancreas, however, is a potentially serious problem; symptoms consist of abdominal discomfort and a gastroenteritis-like illness. Although a polyneuritis and a transverse myelitis have been described, the most common manifestation of CNS infection with varicella is acute cerebellar ataxia. While chickenpox is usually a benign illness in children, other complications such as myocarditis, iritis, nephritis, orchitis, and hepatitis may occur. Pneumonitis occurs more commonly in adults than children.

It can be difficult to distinguish between the vesicular lesions of smallpox and chickenpox. Classically, however, a history of rash with vesicles that develop over a few hours would be typical of a chickenpox infection; vesiculation that develops over a period of days is the rule in smallpox. While fever is characteristic of the prodrome of smallpox, it subsides prior to focal eruptions. Lesions of smallpox are typically all at the same stage of development, in contrast to the various stages seen in a patient with chickenpox. Preparations of vesicular fluid under electron microscopy show characteristic brick-shaped particles with poxvirus. A more readily available test, the Tzanck smear, performed by scraping the base of the lesion, should reveal multinucleated giant cells microscopically in a patient with chickenpox. Humoral immunity appears to be very important in the recovery from enteroviral infections. One of the most common complications for patients with sex-linked or acquired agammaglobulinemia is a chronic central nervous system infection with an echovirus. In the absence of the ability to produce antibodies, this virus spreads rapidly and usually produces a fatal illness. The administration of intravenous preparations of gamma globulin intraventricularly has controlled this serious complication of immune deficiency in some patients.

It may take from 9 to 11 days for the first symptoms of measles to develop after exposure. Malaise, irritability, and a high fever often associated with conjunctivitis with prominent tearing are common symptoms. This prodromal syndrome may last from three days to a week before the characteristic rash of measles develops. One or two days before the onset of the rash, characteristic Koplik's spots—small, red, irregular lesions with blue-white centers—may be visible on the mucous membranes and occasionally on the conjunctiva. Classically, the measles rash will begin on the forehead and spread downward, and the Koplik's spots will rapidly resolve.

42–46. The answers are 42-a, 43-d, 44-b, 45-e, 46-c. *(Sande, 6/e, pp 305–331, 379–399, 207–208, 429–430.)* Pneumonia due to *P. carinii* was among the first recognized manifestations of AIDS. The chest radiograph typically shows a diffuse bilateral interstitial pattern, but other patterns, including a normal radiograph, may occur. *Pneumocystis* infection may also occur at extrapulmonary sites.

Cytomegalovirus (CMV) is a frequent disseminated pathogen that causes retinitis that may lead to blindness. CMV may also cause pneumonitis, adrenalitis, and hepatitis, as well as colitis with significant diarrhea.

The protozoa *Cryptosporidium* may cause a chronic diarrhea that leads to malabsorption and wasting. It can be diagnosed by direct examination of the stool with special concentration or staining techniques or both.

Salmonella infections have been recognized with increased frequency in patients with HIV. These patients are typically bacteremic and develop bacteremic relapse; they do not usually present with a diarrheal illness.

Patients who present with seizures warrant an evaluation for toxoplasmosis. CNS lymphoma and certain other infections may also cause seizures. Patients with toxoplasmic encephalitis may also have toxoplasmic chorioretinitis, although CMV remains the most common identified cause of retinitis in patients with AIDS.

47–51. The answers are 47-c, 48-b, 49-e, 50-d, 51-a. *(Stobo, 23/e, pp 590–603.)* Treatment of gonococcal infections should be guided by the increasing frequency of antibiotic-resistant *Neisseria gonorrhoeae* and high frequency of co-infection with *Chlamydia trachomatis.* Because of the increased frequency of resistance to penicillin and tetracyclines, ceftriaxone is recommended as the treatment of choice. Doxycycline is added to treat chlamydial and other causes of nongonococcal urethritis. First episodes of genital herpes may be particularly severe. Oral acyclovir will accelerate the healing but will not reduce the risk of recurrence once the drug is stopped.

Trichomoniasis is usually diagnosed by a wet preparation microscopic examination or by culture. Both the patient and sexual partner should be treated with metronidazole.

Penicillin remains the drug of choice for treatment of syphilis. The route of administration and duration of therapy depend on the stage of disease and presence of CNS involvement and may also be influenced by the HIV-serostatus of the patient.

52–55. The answers are 52-c, 53-a, 54-a, 55-b. *(Fauci, 14/e, pp 865–867.)* The tetracyclines are associated with photosensitization, and patients taking these antibiotics should be warned about exposure to the sun.

Imipenem, a carbapenem, may cause central nervous system toxicity such as seizures, especially when administered at high dosages.

The major toxicity of gentamicin, an aminoglycoside, is acute tubular necrosis; thus, drug levels should be closely monitored. The aminoglycosides may be ototoxic, with effects on vestibular or auditory function or both. This class of drugs can also produce neuromuscular blockade, especially when administered with concomitant neuromuscular blocking agents or to patients with impairment of neuromuscular transmission, such as myasthenia gravis.

56. The answer is d. *(Fauci, 14/e, pp 1086–1087.)* Varicella pneumonia develops in about 20% of adults with chickenpox. It occurs three to seven days after the onset of the rash. The hallmark of the chickenpox rash is papules, vesicles, and scabs in various stages of development. Fever, malaise, and itching are usually part of the clinical picture. The differential can include some coxsackie and echovirus infection, which might present with pneumonia and vesicular rash. Rickettsialpox, a rickettsial infection, has also been mistaken for chickenpox.

57. The answer is c. *(Stobo, 23/e, pp 605–607.)* Patients with *P. carinii* pneumonia frequently present with shortness of breath and no sputum production. The interstitial pattern of infiltrates on chest x-ray distinguishes the pneumonia from most bacterial infections. Diagnosis is made by review of silver methenamine stain. Serology is not sensitive or specific enough for routine use. The organism does not grow on any media. Cavitation can occur but is quite unusual. The history is likely to suggest a risk factor for HIV disease.

58. The answer is b. *(Gantz, 4/e, pp 455–459.)* Trimethoprim-sulfa is the drug of choice for *P. carinii* pneumonia in the nonallergic patient. Oral therapy is recommended for mild to moderate disease. Prednidone has been shown to improve the mortality rate in moderate to severe disease when the P_{O_2} is less than 70 mm Hg. Neither tetracycline nor erythromycin have any activity to the organism.

59. The answer is c. *(Fauci, 14/e, pp 1045–1047.)* The rash of Rocky Mountain spotted fever occurs about five days into an illness characterized by fever, malaise, and headache. The rash may be macular or petechial, but almost always spreads from the ankles and wrists to the trunk. The disease is most common in spring and summer. North Carolina and East Tennessee have a relatively high index of disease. RMSF is a rickettsial disease with the tick as the vector. About 80% of patients will give a history of tick exposure.

60. The answer is c. *(Fauci, 14/e, pp 828–829.)* The cellulitis described, erysipelas, is typical of infection caused by *Streptococcus pyogenes*–group A beta-hemolytic streptococci. There is often a preceding event such as a cut in the skin, dermatitis, or superficial fungal infection that precedes this rapidly spreading cellulitis. Anaerobic cellulitis is more often associated with underlying diabetes. *Staphylococcus epidermidis* does not cause rapidly progressive cellulitis. *Staphylococcus aureus* can cause cellulitis that is difficult to distinguish from erysipelas, but it is usually more focal and likely to produce furuncles, or abscesses.

61. The answer is c. *(Fauci, 14/e, pp 803–804.)* About half of all cases of nongonococcal urethritis are caused by *Chlamydia trachomatis. Ureaplasma urealyticum* and *Trichomonas vaginalis* are rarer causes of urethritis. Herpes simplex would present with vesicular lesions and pain. *Chlamydia psittaci* is the etiologic agent in psittacosis.

62–68. The answers are 62-a, 63-e, 64-b, 65-c, 66-h, 67-f, 68-j. *(Gorbach, 2/e, pp 1334–1335, 2164–2168, 2327–2329, 2094–2095, 2142, 592, 2314–2315.)* There are several causes for dysphagia in the HIV-positive patient, including *C. albicans*, herpes simplex, and cytomegalovirus. The biopsy result in this patient confirms *Candida* infection with the typical picture of both yeast and hyphae seen on smear. Herpes simplex encephalitis can occur in patients of any age and usually, in immunocompetent patients. The bizarre behavior includes personality aberrations, hypersexuality, or sensory hallucinations. CSF shows lymphocytes with a close to normal sugar and protein. Focal abnormalities are seen in the temporal lobe by CT scan, MRI, or EEG.

The patient who has had a previous history of tuberculosis and now complains of hemoptysis would be reevaluated for active tuberculosis. However, the chest x-ray described is characteristic of a fungus ball—almost always the result of an aspergilloma.

The Filipino patient who has developed a pulmonary nodule after travel through the Southwest would be suspected of having developed coccidioidomycosis. Individuals from the Philippines have a higher incidence of the disease and are more likely to have complications of dissemination.

The 35-year-old with cough, sore throat, and fever went on to develop symptoms of myocarditis with typical ECG findings. Coxsackie B infection is the most likely organism to produce URI symptoms that evolve into a picture of myocarditis. Myocarditis may be asymptomatic or can present with chest pain, both pleuritic and ischemic-like.

Hantavirus pulmonary syndrome begins with a prodromal illness of cough, fever, and myalgias that is difficult to distinguish from other viral illnesses such as influenza. However, the illness progresses to increased dyspnea, hypoxia, and hypotension. The picture resembles adult respiratory distress syndrome, and most patients require mechanical ventilation. Exposure to the deer mouse has been documented in some cases.

The slapped-cheek appearance in the child described, previously called fifth disease, is now known to be the result of a parvovirus B19. Its occurrence may be epidemic in nature. Children are usually not very ill, but adults can develop a polyarthralgia or true arthritis.

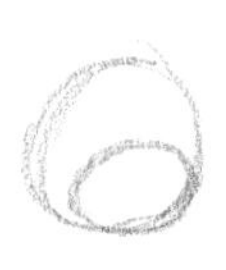

RHEUMATOLOGY

DIRECTIONS: Each item below contains a question or incomplete statement followed by suggested responses. Select the **one best** response to each question.

Items 69–70

69. A 40-year-old female complains of seven weeks of pain and swelling in both wrists and knees. The patient complained of fatigue and lethargy several weeks before noticing the joint pain. The patient notes that after a period of rest, resistance to movement is more striking. On exam the metacarpophalangeal joints and wrists are warm and tender. There are no other joint abnormalities. There is no alopecia, photosensitivity, kidney disease, or rash. Which of the following is correct?

a. The clinical picture suggests early rheumatoid arthritis, and a rheumatoid factor should be obtained
b. The prodrome of lethargy suggests chronic fatigue syndrome
c. Lack of systemic symptoms suggests osteoarthritis
d. X-rays of the hand are likely to show joint-space narrowing and erosion

70. On follow-up, over several months the patient continues to complain of joint stiffness. In addition to swelling of the wrist and MCPs, tenderness and joint effusion has occurred in both knees. The rheumatoid factor has become positive and subcutaneous nodules are noted on the extensor surfaces of the forearm. Which of the following statements is correct?

a. Corticosteroids should be started
b. The patient meets the American College of Rheumatology criteria for RA and should be evaluated by a rheumatologist for disease modifying antirheumatic therapy
c. A nonsteroidal anti-inflammatory drug should be added to aspirin
d. The patient's prognosis is highly favorable

71. A 60-year-old female complains of dry mouth and a gritty sensation in her eyes. It is sometimes difficult to speak for more than a few minutes. There is no history of diabetes mellitus and no history of neurologic disease. The patient is on no medications. On exam the buccal mucosa appears dry, and the salivary glands are enlarged bilaterally. The next step in evaluation would be

a. Lip biopsy
b. Schirmer test and measurement of autoantibodies
c. IgG antibody to mumps virus
d. Use of corticosteroids

72. A 40-year-old male complains of exquisite pain and tenderness over the left ankle. There is no history of trauma. The patient is taking a mild diuretic for hypertension. On exam, the ankle is very swollen and tender. There are no other physical exam abnormalities. The next step in management is

a. Begin colchicine and broad-spectrum antibiotics
b. Obtain uric acid level and perform arthrocentesis
c. Begin allopurinol if uric acid level is elevated
d. Obtain ankle x-ray to rule out fracture

Items 73–74

73. A 70-year-old male complains of fever and pain in his left knee. Several days previously, the patient skinned his knee while working in his garage. He is not sexually active. The knee is red, warm, and swollen. An arthocentesis is performed, which shows 200,000 leukocytes/mm^3, a protein of 3 g/dL, and a glucose of 20 mg/dL. No crystals are noted. The most important next step would be

a. Gram stain and culture of joint fluid
b. Urethral culture
c. Uric acid level
d. Antinuclear antibody

74. The most likely organism to cause septic arthritis in the case above is

a. *Streptococcus pneumoniae*
b. *Neisseria gonorrhoeae*
c. *Escherichia coli*
d. *Staphylococcus aureus*

75. A 50-year-old male complains of low back pain and stiffness, which becomes worse on bending and is relieved by lying down. There are no symptoms of fever, chills, weight loss, or urinary problems. He has had similar pain several years ago. On exam there is paraspinal tenderness and spasm of the lower lumbar back. There are no sensory deficits, and reflexes are normal. The next step in management would be

a. Lumbosacral spine films
b. Stretching exercises
c. Weight training
d. Bed rest with pain control
e. MRI

76. A 60-year-old male complains of pain in both knees coming on gradually over the past two years. The pain is relieved by rest and worsened by the movement. There is bony enlargement of the knees with mild inflammation. Crepitation is noted on motion of the knee joint. There are no other findings except for bony enlargement at the distal interphalangeal joint. The patient is 5 feet 9 inches tall and weighs 190 pounds. The best way to prevent disease progression is

a. Weight reduction
b. Calcium supplementation
c. Total knee replacement
d. Aspirin
e. Prednisone orally

77. A 22-year-old male develops the insidious onset of low back pain improved with exercise and worsened by rest. There is no history of diarrhea, conjunctivitis, urethritis, eye problems, or nail changes. On exam the patient has loss of mobility with respect to lumbar flexion and extension. He has a kyphotic posture. A plain film of the spine shows widening and sclerosis of the sacroiliac joints. Some calcification is noted in the anterior spinal ligament. Which of the following best characterizes this patient's disease process?

a. He is most likely to have acute lumbosacral back strain and requires bed rest
b. The patient has a spondyloarthropathy, most likely ankylosing spondylitis
c. The patient is likely to die from pulmonary fibrosis and extrathoracic restrictive lung disease
d. A rheumatoid factor is likely to be positive
e. A colonoscopy is likely to show Crohn's disease

78. A 20-year-old woman has developed low-grade fever, a malar rash, and arthralgias of the hands over several months. High titers of anti-DNA antibodies are noted and complement levels are low. The patient's white blood cell count is 3000/mm^3 and platelet count is 90,000/mm^3. The patient is on no medications and has no signs of active infection. Which of the following statements is correct?

a. If glomerulonephritis, severe thrombocytopenia, or hemolytic anemia develops, high-dose glucocorticoid therapy would be indicated
b. Central nervous system symptoms will occur within 10 years
c. The patient can be expected to develop Raynaud's phenomenon when exposed to cold
d. The patient will have a false-positive test for syphillis
e. The disease process described is an absolute contraindication to pregnancy

79. A 45-year-old woman has pain in her fingers on exposure to cold, arthralgias, and difficulty swallowing solid food. The most useful test to make a definitive diagnosis would be

a. Rheumatoid factor
b. Antinucleolar antibody
c. ECG
d. BUN and creatinine

80. A 20-year-old male complains of arthritis and eye irritation. He has a history of burning on urination. On exam there is a joint effusion of the right knee and a dermatitis of the glans penis. Which of the following is correct?

a. *N. gonorrhoeae* is likely to be cultured from the glans penis
b. The patient is likely to be rheumatoid-factor-positive
c. An infectious process of the GI tract may precipitate this disease
d. An ANA is very likely to be positive

Items 81–82

81. A 75-year-old male complains of unilateral headache. On one occasion he transiently lost his vision. He also complains of aching in the shoulders and neck. There are no focal neurologic findings. Carotid pulses are normal without bruit. There is some tenderness over the left temple. Laboratory data shows a mild anemia. Which of the following tests is most likely to be abnormal?

a. Carotid ultrasound
b. CT scan
c. Erythrocyte sedimentation rate
d. X-ray left shoulder
e. Skull films

82. In the above patient, who is shown to have an elevated ESR, the best approach to management would be

a. Begin glucocorticoid therapy and arrange for temporal artery biopsy
b. Schedule biopsy and begin corticosteroids based on biopsy results and clinical course
c. Schedule carotid angiography
d. Follow ESR and consider further studies if it remains elevated

Items 83–84

83. A 65-year-old male developed the sudden onset of severe knee pain. The knee is red, swollen, and tender. He has a history of diabetes mellitus and cardiomyopathy. An x-ray of the knee shows linear calcification. Definitive diagnosis is best made by

a. Serum uric acid
b. Serum calcium
c. Arthrocentesis and identification of positive birefringent rhomboid crystals
d. Rheumatoid factor

84. Further workup in this patient should include evaluation for

a. Renal disease
b. Hemochromatosis
c. Peptic ulcer disease
d. Lyme disease

85. A 35-year-old woman complains of aching all over. She sleeps poorly and all her joints hurt. Symptoms have progressed over several years. Physical exam shows multiple points of tenderness over the neck, shoulders, elbows, and wrists. There is no joint swelling or deformity. A complete blood count and erythrocyte sedimentation rate are normal. Rheumatoid factor is negative. There is no tenderness over the median third of the clavicle, the medial malleolus, or the forehead. The best therapeutic option in this patient is

a. Amytriptyline at night
b. Prednisone
c. Aspirin and methotrexate
d. Plaquenil

86. A 70-year-old female with mild dementia complains of hip pain. There is some limitation of motion in the right hip. The first step in evaluation would be

a. CBC and erythrocyte sedimentation rate
b. Rheumatoid factor
c. X-ray of right hip
d. Bone scan

DIRECTIONS: Each group of questions below consists of lettered headings followed by a set of numbered items. For each numbered item select the **one** lettered heading with which it is most closely associated. Each lettered heading may be used once, more than once, or not at all.

Items 87–90

Select the most probable diagnosis for each patient.

a. Behçet's syndrome
b. Ankylosing spondylitis
c. Polymyalgia rheumatica
d. Reiter's syndrome
e. Drug-induced lupus erythematosus
f. Polyarteritis nodosa
g. Scleroderma

87. A 50-year-old drug abuser presents with fever, weight loss. Exam shows hypertension, nodular skin rash, peripheral neuropathy; ESR is 100 mm/L; RBC casts seen on urine analysis.

88. An elderly male presents with pain in shoulders and hands. ESR is 105 mm/L. History includes transient blindness and unilateral headache.

89. A young male presents with leg swelling and recurrent aphthous ulcers of lips and tongue. Has also recently noted painful genital ulcers. No urethritis or conjunctivitis. On exam he has evidence of deep vein thrombophlebitis.

90. A 19-year-old male complains of low back morning stiffness, pain and limitation of motion of shoulders. Has eye pain and photophobia. Diastolic murmur is present on physical exam.

Items 91–93

For each finding, select the most appropriate diagnosis.

a. Rheumatoid arthritis
b. Psoriatic arthritis
c. Ankylosing spondylitis
d. Reiter's syndrome
e. Behçet's syndrome
f. Disseminated gonococcemia
g. Paget's disease

91. Proximal and distal interphalangeal joints are most frequently involved. Nails may show pitting or onycholysis.

92. Recurrent aphthous ulcers. Painful genital lesions. Tenderness of knees without deformity.

93. Conjunctivitis, balanitis, monarthritis. Hyperkeratotic lesions on soles of feet. Antecedent diarrhea one week before symptoms.

DIRECTIONS: The item below contains a question or incomplete statement followed by suggested responses. Select the **one best** response to the question.

94. A 65-year-old woman who has a 12-year history of symmetrical polyarthritis is admitted to the hospital. Physical examination reveals splenomegaly, ulcerations over the lateral malleoli, and synovitis of the wrists, shoulders, and knees. There is no hepatomegaly. Laboratory values demonstrate a white blood cell count of 2500/mm^3 and a rheumatoid factor titer of 1:4096. This patient's white blood cell differential count is likely to reveal

a. Pancytopenia
b. Lymphopenia
c. Granulocytopenia
d. Lymphocytosis
e. Basophilia

DIRECTIONS: Each group of questions below consists of lettered headings followed by a set of numbered items. For each numbered item select the **one** lettered heading with which it is most closely associated. Each lettered heading may be used once, more than once, or not at all.

Items 95–99

For each condition, select the drug with which it is closely associated.

a. Acetylsalicylic acid (aspirin)
b. Gold
c. Prednisone
d. Chloroquine
e. None of the above

95. Gastrointestinal bleeding

96. Osteoporosis

97. Retinopathy

98. Proteinuria

99. Stomatitis

Items 100–104

Match each description with the appropriate disease.

a. Polyarteritis nodosa
b. Wegener's granulomatosis
c. Giant cell arteritis
d. Multiple cholesterol embolization syndrome
e. Takayasu's arteritis

100. Involvement of the upper and lower respiratory tracts; a cause of glomerulonephritis

101. Ecchymoses and necrosis in extremities in elderly patients

102. Inflammation of small- to medium-size muscular arteries, which may cause kidney, heart, liver, gastrointestinal, and muscular damage

103. Patients above the age of 55, who may experience fever, weight loss, scalp pain, headache, and visual changes

104. Inflammation of the aorta and its branches in young women; also known as *pulseless disease*

Items 105–107

For each numbered item below, select the most likely disease process.

a. Gonococcal arthritis
b. Reiter's syndrome
c. Behçet's syndrome
d. Churg-Strauss syndrome
e. Temporal arteritis

105. Autoimmune disease in patient HLA-B27-positive

106. Positive for antineutrophil cytoplasmic antibody

107. Circulating autoantibodies to human oral mucous membrane

RHEUMATOLOGY

Answers

69. The answer is a. *(Stobo, 23/e, pp 204–214.)* The clinical picture of symmetrical swelling and tenderness of the metacarpophalangeal (MCP) and wrist joints lasting longer than six weeks strongly suggests rheumatoid arthritis. Rheumatoid factor, an immunoglobulin directed against the Fc portion of IgG, is positive in about 80% of cases and is present early in the disease. The history of lethargy or fatigue is a common prodrome of RA. The inflammatory joint changes are not consistent with chronic fatigue syndrome. The MCP/wrist distribution of joint symptoms makes osteoarthritis very unlikely. The x-ray changes described are characteristic of RA, but would occur later in the course of the disease.

70. The answer is b. *(Stobo, 23/e, pp 204–214.)* The patient has more than four of the required signs or symptoms of RA, including morning stiffness, swelling of wrist or MCP, simultaneous swelling of joints on both sides of body, subcutaneous nodules, and positive rheumatoid factor. Subcutaneous nodules are a poor prognostic sign for the activity of the disease. A rheumatologist should be consulted and disease-modifying drugs (gold, penicillamine, antimalarials, or methotrexate) should be instituted. Corticosteroids are generally withheld unless absolutely necessary and after disease-modifying drugs are instituted. There is no value to using both aspirin and nonsteroidals together. Simultaneous usage will increase side effects.

71. The answer is b. *(Stobo, 23/e, pp 211–214.)* The complaints described are characteristic of Sjögren's syndrome, an autoimmune disease with presenting symptoms of dry eyes and dry mouth. The disease is caused by lymphocytic infiltration and destruction of lacrimal and salivary glands. Dry eyes can be measured objectively by Schirmer's test, which measures the amount of wetness of a piece of filter paper when exposed to the lower lid for five minutes. Most patients with Sjögren's produce autoantibodies, particularly anti-RO (SSA). Lip biopsy is needed only to evaluate uncertain cases such as when dry mouth occurs without dry eye symptoms. Mumps can cause bilateral parotitis, but would not explain the patient's dry eye syndrome. Corticosteroids are reserved for life-threatening vasculitis, which may cause a secondary Sjögren's syndrome.

72. The answer is b. *(Stobo, 23/e, pp 233–239.)* The sudden onset and severity of this monoarticular arthritis suggests acute gouty arthritis, especially in a patient on diuretic therapy. However, an arthocentesis is indicated in the first episode to document gout by demonstrating needle-shaped, negatively birefringent crystals and to rule out other diagnosis such as infection. For most patients with acute gout, NSAIDs are the treatment of choice. Colchicine is also effective, but causes nausea and diarrhea. Antibiotics should not be started for infectious arthritis before an arthrocentesis is performed. Hyperuricemia should never be treated in the setting of an acute attack of gouty arthritis. X-ray of the ankle would likely be inconclusive in this patient with no trauma history.

73. The answer is a. *(Stobo, 23/e, pp 251–256.)* The clinical and laboratory picture suggests an acute septic arthritis. The most important first step is to determine the etiologic agent of the infection. Gout would be unlikely to produce the 200,000 leukocytes in the joint fluid. There is no history of symptoms suggesting connective tissue disease. Gonococci can cause a septic arthritis, but a urethral culture in the absence of urethral discharge would not be helpful.

74. The answer is d. *(Stobo, 23/e, pp 251–256.)* *S. aureus* is the most common organism to cause septic arthritis in adults. Beta-hemolytic streptococci are the second most common. *N. gonorrhoeae* can also produce septic arthritis, but would be less likely in this patient who is not sexually active. *S. pneumoniae* and *E. coli* are rare causes of septic arthritis and usually occur secondary to a primary focus of infection.

75. The answer is d. *(Stobo, 23/e, pp 261–265.)* The patient presents with symptoms consistent with acute mechanical low back pain. Even patients with lumbar disc herniation and sciatica improve with nonoperative care, and imaging studies do not affect initial management. Bed rest, three to seven days, is recommended, with adequate pain control and reassurance. Active therapy to restore range of motion and function is appropriate after pain and spasm are relieved.

76. The answer is a. *(Stobo, 23/e, pp 240–244.)* The clinical picture of a noninflammatory arthritis of weight-bearing joints is suggestive of degenerative joint disease, also called *osteoarthritis.* Crepitation over the involved joints is characteristic, as are the bony enlargements of the DIP joints. In this overweight patient, weight reduction is the best method to decrease the risk of further degenerative changes. Aspirin can be used as symptomatic treatment, but does not affect the course of the disease. Calcium supplementation may be relevant to associated osteoporosis, but not to the osteoarthritis. Oral prednisone would be contraindicated; intraarticular corticosteroid injections may be given once or twice per year for symptom reduction, but will accelerate damage to cartilage. Knee replacement is the treatment of last resort, usually when pain occurs around the clock and symptoms are not controlled by medical regimens.

77. The answer is b. *(Stobo, 23/e, pp 227–233.)* Insidious back pain occurring in a young male that improves with exercise suggests one of the spondyloarthropathies—ankylosing spondylitis, Reiter's, psoriatic arthritis, or enteropathic arthritis. Ankylosing spondylitis is most likely in this patient. Acute lumbosacral strain would not be relieved by exercise or worsened by rest. The prognosis in ankylosing spondylitis is generally very good, with only 6% dying of the disease itself. While pulmonary fibrosis and restrictive lung disease can occur, it is rarely a cause of death (cervical fracture, heart block, and amyloidosis are leading causes of death in ankylosing spondylitis). Rheumatoid factor is negative in all the spondyloarthropathies. Crohn's disease can cause an enteropathic arthritis, but without gastrointestinal symptoms, this diagnosis is unlikely.

78. The answer is a. *(Stobo, 23/e, pp 197–203.)* The combination of fever, malar rash, and arthralgias suggests systemic lupus erythematosus, and the patient's thrombocytopenia, leukopenia, and positive antibody to native DNA provide more than four criteria for a definitive diagnosis. High-dose corticosteroids would therefore be indicated for any life-threatening complication of lupus such as described in item a. Patients with SLE have an unpredictable course. No patients develop all signs or symptoms. Neuropsychiatric disease occurs at some time in about half of all SLE patients and Raynaud's phenomenon in about 25%. Pregnancy is relatively safe in women with SLE who have controlled disease and are on less than 10 mg of prednisone.

79. The answer is b. *(Stobo, 23/e, pp 245–251.)* The symptoms of Raynaud's phenomenon, arthralgia, and dysphagia point toward the diagnosis of sclerodema. Antinuclear antibody occurs in only 20% of patients with the disease, but a positive test is highly specific. Cardiac involvement may occur, and an ECG could show heart block or pericardial involvement. Renal failure can develop insidiously. Rheumatoid factor is nonspecific and present in about 20% of patients with sclerodema.

80. The answer is c. *(Stobo, 23/e, p 230.)* Reiter's syndrome is characterized as a triad of oligoarticular arthritis, conjunctivitis, and urethritis. The disease is often precipitated by bacterial diarrhea. ANA and rheumatoid factor are usually negative. Gonorrhea can precipitate Reiter's syndrome, but patients with the disease are culture-negative.

81. The answer is c. *(Stobo, 23/e, pp 217–218.)* Unilateral headache and visual loss in this elderly patient with polymyalgia rheumatica symptoms lead to a clinical diagnosis of temporal arteritis. The erythrocyte sedimentation rate is high in almost all of these patients. Skull x-ray and CT scan would be normal. Carotid disease would not be expected.

82. The answer is a. *(Stobo, 23/e, pp 217–218.)* Biopsy results should not delay corticosteroid therapy. Biopsies may show vasculitis even after 14 days of glucocorticoid therapy. Delay risks loss of sight permanently. Once an episode of loss of vision occurs, workup must proceed as quickly as possible.

83. The answer is c. *(Stobo, 23/e, pp 238–239.)* The acute monoarticular arthritis in association with linear calcification of the cartilage of the knee suggests the diagnosis of pseudogout, also called *calcium pyrophosphate dihydrate deposition* disease. The disease resembles gout. Positive birefringent crystals can be demonstrated in joint fluid. Serum uric acid and calcium levels are normal, as is the rheumatoid factor.

84. The answer is b. *(Stobo, 23/e, pp 238–239.)* Pseudogout may be associated with hemochromatosis. Since the patient has a history of diabetes mellitus and cardiomyopathy, this process must be considered. Serum ferritin and serum iron saturation should be measured.

85. The answer is a. *(Fauci, 14/e, pp 1955–1956.)* The patient's multiple trigger points, associated sleep disturbance, and lack of joint or muscle findings makes fibromyalgia a possible diagnosis. The diagnosis hinges on the multiple tender points. CBC and ESR are characteristically normal. Tricyclic antidepressants restore sleep; aspirin and other anti-inflammatory drugs are not helpful. Biofeedback and exercise programs have been partially successful. The clavicle, medial malleolus, and forehead are never trigger points for the process.

86. The answer is c. *(Stein, 5/e, p 2290.)* A film of the right hip is mandatory in this patient. Fracture of the hip must be ruled out, particularly in a woman with mental status abnormalities, who may be prone to falls.

87–90. The answers are 87-f, 88-c, 89-a, 90-b. *(Fauci, 14/e, pp 1910, 1904–1906, 1917, 1912–1913.)* Behçet's syndrome is a multisystem disorder that usually presents with recurrent oral and genital ulcers. One-fourth of patients develop superficial or deep vein thrombophlebitis. Iritis, uveitis, and nondeforming arthritis may also occur.

The 50-year-old drug abuser also has a multisystem disease, including systemic complaints, hypertension, skin lesions, neuropathy, and an abnormal urine sediment. This complex suggests a vasculitis, particularly polyarteritis nodosa, and 20 to 30% of patients have hepatitis B antigenemia. The disease is a necrotizing vasculitis of small and medium muscular arteries. The pathology of the kidney includes an arteritis and, in some cases, a glomerulitis. Nodular skin lesions show vasculitis on biopsy. The 19-year-old with low back pain, morning stiffness, and eye pain has complaints that suggest ankylosing spondylitis. This is an inflammatory disorder that affects the axial skeleton. It is an autoimmune disorder that has a close association with HLA B27 histocompatibility antigen. Anterior uveitis is the most common extraarticular complaint. Aortic regurgitation occurs in a few percent of patients.

The elderly male presents with nonspecific joint complaints typical of polymyalgia rheumatica. The high erythrocyte sedimentation rate is characteristic. The transient loss of vision suggests concomitant temporal arteritis, an important association seen particularly in older patients.

91–93. The answers are 91-b, 92-e, 93-d. *(Fauci, 14/e, pp 1949–1950, 1910, 1060.)* Psoriatic arthritis is a chronic inflammatory process. Psoriatic arthritis most frequently involves the proximal and distal interphalangeal joints. Knees, hips, and ankles may also be involved. Nail abnormalities are common and may include ridging or pitting of nails as well as onycholysis.

Arthritis that occurs in association with aphthous ulcers and genital lesions is a clinical clue to Behçet's syndrome. This is a multisystem disorder, an autoimmune disease that results in vasculitis. Painful, recurrent aphthous ulcers come and go in the oral mucosa. Ulcers may be shallow or deep and occur singly or in crops. Genital ulcers have an appearance similar to the oral lesions. The arthritis of Behçet's syndrome is nondeforming and usually involves the knees and ankles.

Reiter's syndrome is a reactive arthritis occurring after certain antecedent infections, including shigella, salmonella, yersinia, and campylobacter; 60 to 85% of patients with Reiter's syndrome have inherited the HLA B27 gene. The syndrome includes transient monarthritis and balanitis (inflammation of the glans penis), with or without urethritis. The lesions described are termed *keratoderma blennorrhagica.* These lesions start as vesicles but become hyperkeratotic. They usually occur on the palms of the hand or on the soles of the feet.

94. The answer is c. *(Fauci, 14/e, p 1884.)* Felty's syndrome consists of a triad of rheumatoid arthritis, splenomegaly, and leukopenia. In contrast to the lymphopenia observed in patients who have systemic lupus erythematosus, the leukopenia of Felty's syndrome is related to a reduction in the number of circulating polymorphonuclear leukocytes. The mechanism of the granulocytopenia is poorly understood. Felty's syndrome tends to occur in people who have had active rheumatoid arthritis for a prolonged period. These patients commonly have other systemic features of rheumatoid disease such as nodules, skin ulcerations, the sicca complex, peripheral sensory and motor neuropathy, and arteritic lesions.

95–99. The answers are 95-a, 96-c, 97-d, 98-b, 99-b. *(Fauci, 14/e, pp 1885–1888.)* Drugs used in the treatment of rheumatoid arthritis are broadly classified as anti-inflammatory or remission-inducing (remittive) agents. Aspirin, a nonsteroidal anti-inflammatory agent that inhibits prostaglandin synthesis, is a commonly used first-line drug. The most frequent side effect is gastrointestinal distress. Gold therapy is effective in many patients with rheumatoid arthritis, especially in those whose disease is of recent onset. Side effects, however, are significant and include a dermatitis that may lead to exfoliative dermatitis if treatment is not discontinued, stomatitis, the nephrotic syndrome, and bone marrow suppression. Patients' response to gold may be only temporary.

Low-dose prednisone may be very useful in controlling an acute flare of arthritis or in controlling the disease while waiting for a remittive agent to begin working. However, prednisone has significant toxicity, including osteoporosis.

The most significant side effect of chloroquine is deposition of the drug in the pigmented layer of the retina. Irreversible retina degeneration may develop, and this has limited the use of this drug. Hydroxychloroquine (Plaquenil) is less frequently associated with retinopathy. Ophthalmic examinations are required every six months during therapy.

100–104. The answers are 100-b, 101-d, 102-a, 103-c, 104-e. *(Fauci, 14/e, pp 1910–1922.)* Wegener's granulomatosis is a granulomatous vasculitis of small arteries and veins that affects the lungs, sinuses, nasopharynx, and the kidneys, where it causes a focal and segmental glomerulonephritis. Other organs can also be damaged, including the skin, eyes, and nervous system. Most patients with the disease develop antibodies to certain proteins in the cytoplasm of neutrophils called *antineutrophil cytoplasmic antibodies* (ANCA).

Elderly people may have extensive atherosclerosis. Especially after an endovascular procedure (like vascular catheterization, grafting, or repair), some of the atheromatous material may embolize, usually to the skin, kidneys, and brain. This material is capable of fixing complement and thus causing vascular damage. The skin lesions—ecchymoses and necrosis—look much like vasculitis. Differentiation between cholesterol embolization and idiopathic vasculitis is important, since not only is the former not steroid-sensitive, but there have been reports of increasing damage after the institution of steroid therapy. Polyarteritis nodosa is a multisystem necrotizing vasculitis that, prior to the use of steroids and cyclophosphamide, was uniformly fatal. In 30% of patients, antecedent hepatitis B virus infection can be demonstrated; immune complexes containing the virus have been found in such patients and are likely pathogenetic.

Giant cell arteritis is a disease of elderly patients that classically affects the temporal arteries (thus the old name, *temporal arteritis*). Giant cell arteritis, named for the presence of giant cells and granulomata that disrupt the internal elastica of the vessel, may present with headache, anemia, a high ESR (although a normal ESR does not rule out the diagnosis), and occasionally a syndrome known as *polymyalgia rheumatica.* This includes stiffness, aching, and tenderness of the proximal muscles. These patients describe weakness of the hip and shoulder girdles, but there is no objective weakness of the muscles, and the muscle enzymes are normal. Giant cell arteritis usually responds to steroid therapy, 45 to 60 mg per day of prednisone; polymyalgia rheumatica typically responds to low-dose prednisone, 10 to 15 mg per day.

First described in Japan and then in Turkey, Takayasu's arteritis is a granulomatous inflammation of the aorta and its main branches. Symptoms are due to local vascular occlusion; aortic regurgitation, systemic and pulmonary hypertension, and general symptoms of arthralgia, fatigue, malaise, anorexia, and weight loss may occur. Surgery may be necessary to correct occlusive lesions.

105–107. The answers are 105-b, 106-d, 107-c. *(Fauci, 14/e, pp 1910, 1914, 1907.)* Reiter's syndrome is characterized as a triad of seronegative, oligoarticular, asymmetrical arthritis; conjunctivitis; and urethritis. The arthritis coupled with urethritis or cervicitis may be sufficient for the diagnosis. It is the most common cause of arthritis in young men. The syndrome develops in up to 3% of males with nongonococcal urethritis, in 2 to 3% of patients with bacillary dysentery, and in 20% of persons with the HLA-B27 antigen. While the pathogenesis is unclear, an infectious process of the urogenital tract (postvenereal Reiter's) or gut (postsdysentery Reiter's) together with a particular genetic background may trigger the development of Reiter's syndrome.

The disorder usually begins with urethritis followed by conjunctivitis, which is usually minimal, and rheumatological findings. The arthritis is usually acute, asymmetrical, and oligoarticular and involves predominantly the joints of the lower extremities; tenosynovitis, dactylitis, and plantar fasciitis also occur. Painless, superficial lesions of the mucosa and glans penis occur in a third of patients; keratosis blennorrhagica occurs in up to 30% of postvenereal Reiter's syndrome patients but does not occur in postdysentery patients; circinate balanitis is a characteristic dermatitis of the glans penis. Churg-Strauss disease is a multiorgan system process caused by granulomatous angiitis. It is similar to polyarteritis nodosa but is more likely to involve the lung. Patients have antineutrophil cytoplasmic antibody of a different type than seen in Wegner's granulomatosis.

Patients with Behçet's syndrome have recurrent, painful aphthus ulcers that are usually deep and located anywhere in the oral cavity. There are frequently concomitant genital ulcers. These patients have a genetic predisposition to the disease and have circulating autoantibodies to oral mucosa membrane in at least 50% of cases.

Pulmonary Disease

DIRECTIONS: Each item below contains a question or incomplete statement followed by suggested responses. Select the **one best** response to each question.

108. A 50-year-old patient with long-standing chronic obstructive lung disease develops the insidious onset of aching in the distal extremities, particularly the wrist bilaterally. There is a 10-pound weight loss. Skin over the wrists is warm and erythematous. There is bilateral clubbing. Plain film is read as "periosteal thickening, possible osteomyelitis." You would

a. Start ciprofloxacin
b. Obtain chest x-ray
c. Aspirate both wrists
d. Begin gold therapy

109. A patient with low-grade fever and weight loss has poor excursion on the right side of the chest, with decreased fremitus, flatness to percussion, and decreased breath sounds all on the right. The trachea is deviated to the left. Likely diagnosis is

a. Pneumothorax
b. Pleural effusion secondary to histoplasmosis
c. Consolidated pneumonia
d. Atelectasis

110. A 60-year-old female with a history of urinary tract infection, steroid-dependent chronic obstructive lung disease, and asthma presents with bilateral infiltrates and an eosinophil count of 15%. The least likely diagnosis is

a. Bronchopulmonary aspergillosis
b. Hypersensitivity pneumonitis
c. Strongyloides hyperinfection syndrome
d. Drug effect of nitrofurantoin

111. A 40-year-old alcoholic develops cough and fever. Chest x-ray shows an air-fluid level in the superior segment of the right lower lobe. The most likely etiologic agent is

a. *S. pneumoniae*
b. *H. influenzae*
c. *Legionella*
d. Anaerobes

DIRECTIONS: Each group of questions below consists of lettered headings followed by a set of numbered items. For each numbered item select the **one** lettered heading with which it is most closely associated. Each lettered heading may be used once, more than once, or not at all.

Items 112–116

Match the disease entity with the type of pleural effusion.

a. pH less than 7.0
b. Right-sided effusion, protein 2.5 g/dL
c. Pleural fluid glucose less than 15 mg/dL
d. Exudate, 100% lymphocytes
e. Bloody effusion
f. Milky appearing
g. Low cholesterol

112. Congestive heart failure

113. Tuberculosis

114. Empyema

115. Rheumatoid arthritis

116. Mesothelioma

Items 117–120

Match the chest x-ray letter with the most likely clinical description.

117. Fever, shaking chills. Sputum Gram stain shows gram-positive cocci in clusters

118. Shortness of breath, awakens gasping for breath at night

119. Fever, night sweats for one year

120. Long-standing hypertension

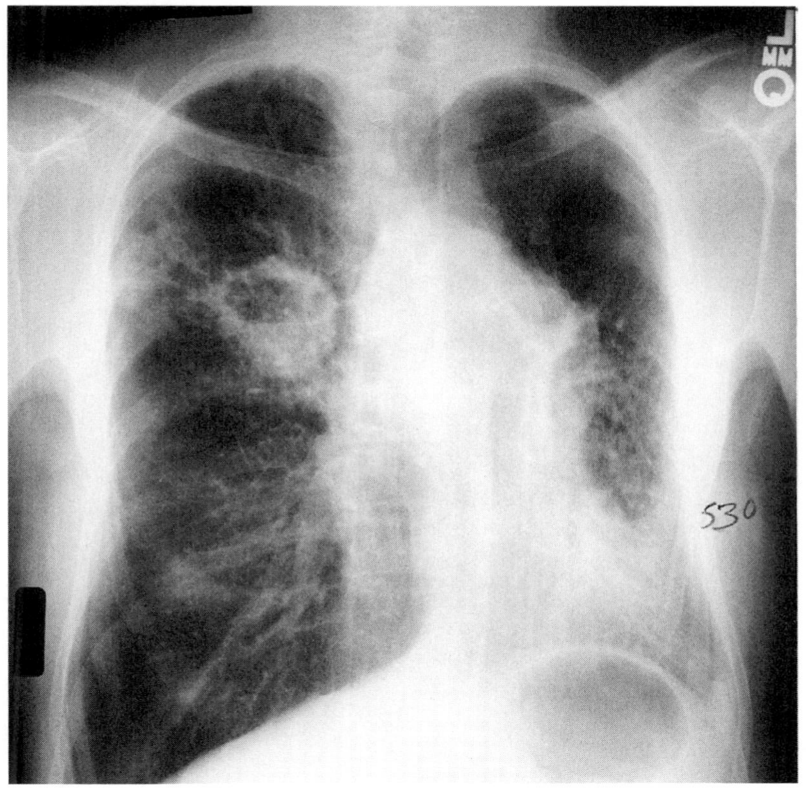

A

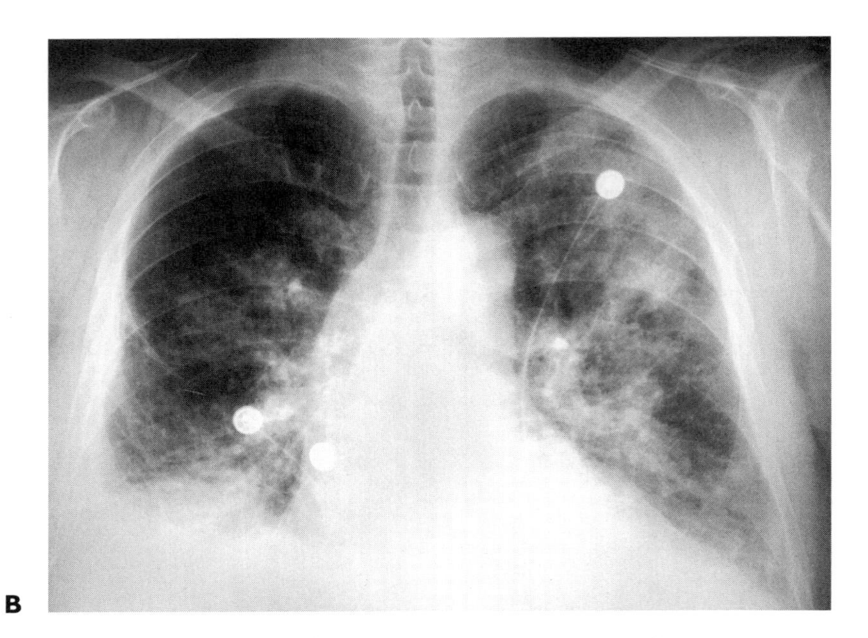

B

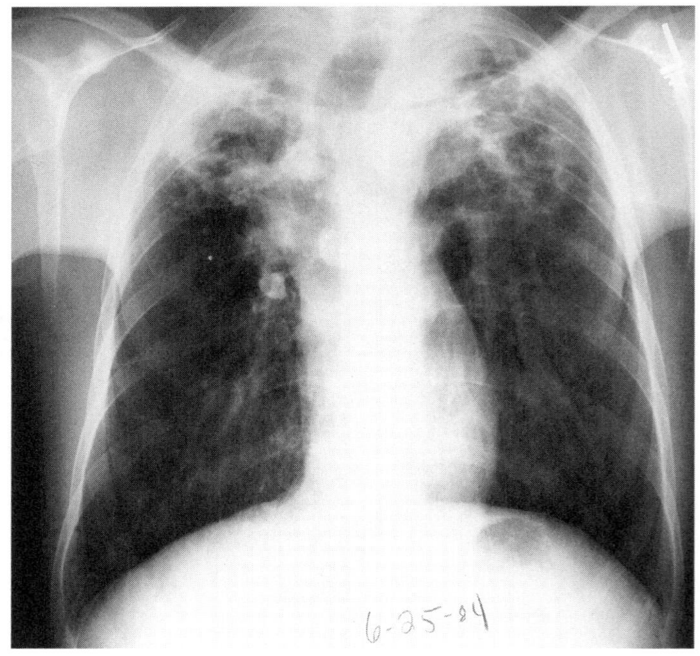

C

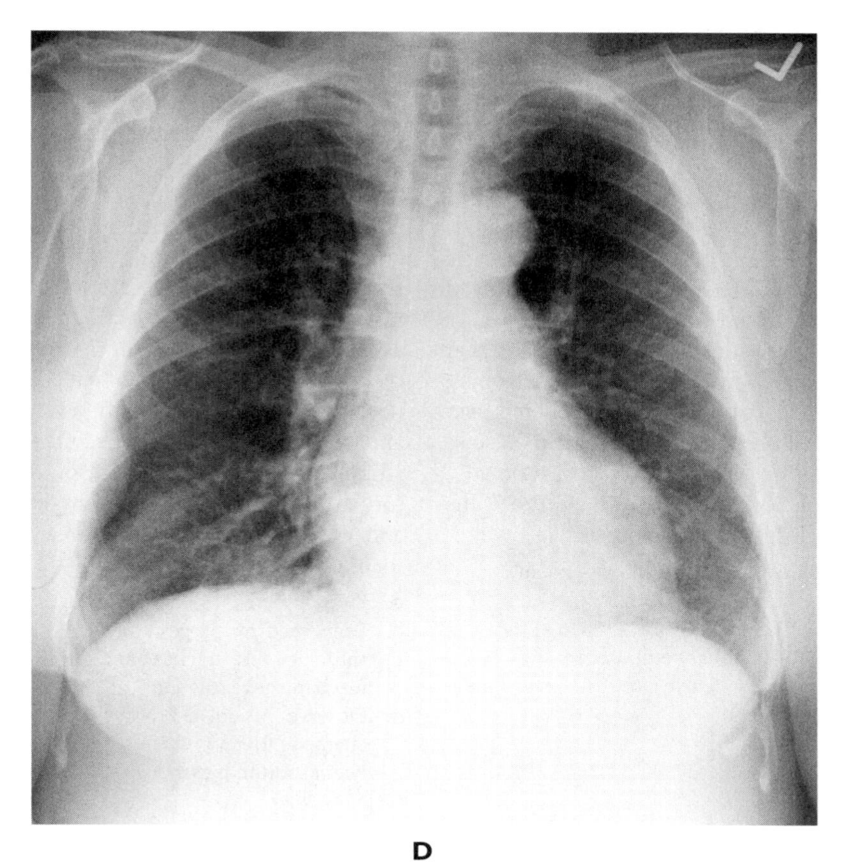

D

DIRECTIONS: Each item below contains a question or incomplete statement followed by suggested responses. Select the **one best** response to each question.

121. A 30-year-old male is admitted to the hospital after a motorcycle accident that resulted in a fracture of the right femur. The fracture is managed with traction. Three days later he becomes confused and tachypneic. A petechial rash is noted over the chest. Lungs are clear to auscultation. Arterial blood gases show P_{O_2} of 50, P_{CO_2} of 28, Ph of 7.49. The most likely diagnosis is

a. Unilateral pulmonary edema
b. Hematoma of chest
c. Fat embolism
d. Pulmonary embolism
e. Early *Staphylococcus aureus* pneumonia

122. A 70-year-old patient with chronic obstructive lung disease requires 2 liters of nasal O_2 to treat his hypoxia, which is sometimes associated with angina. While receiving nasal O_2, the patient develops pleuritic chest pain, fever, and purulent sputum. He becomes stuporous and develops a respiratory acidosis with CO_2 retention and worsening hypoxia. The treatment of choice would be

a. Stop oxygen
b. Begin medroxyprogesterone
c. Intubate the trachea and begin mechanical ventilation
d. Observe patient 24 hours before changing therapy
e. Begin sodium bicarbonate

123. A 34-year-old black female presents to your office with symptoms of cough, dyspnea, and lymphadenopathy. Physical exam shows cervical adenopathy and hepatomegaly. Her chest radiograph is shown in the illustration below. How would you pursue diagnosis?

a. Open-lung biopsy
b. Liver biopsy
c. Bronchoscopy and transbronchial lung biopsy
d. Scalene-node biopsy
e. Obtain a serum angiotensin-converting (ACE) level

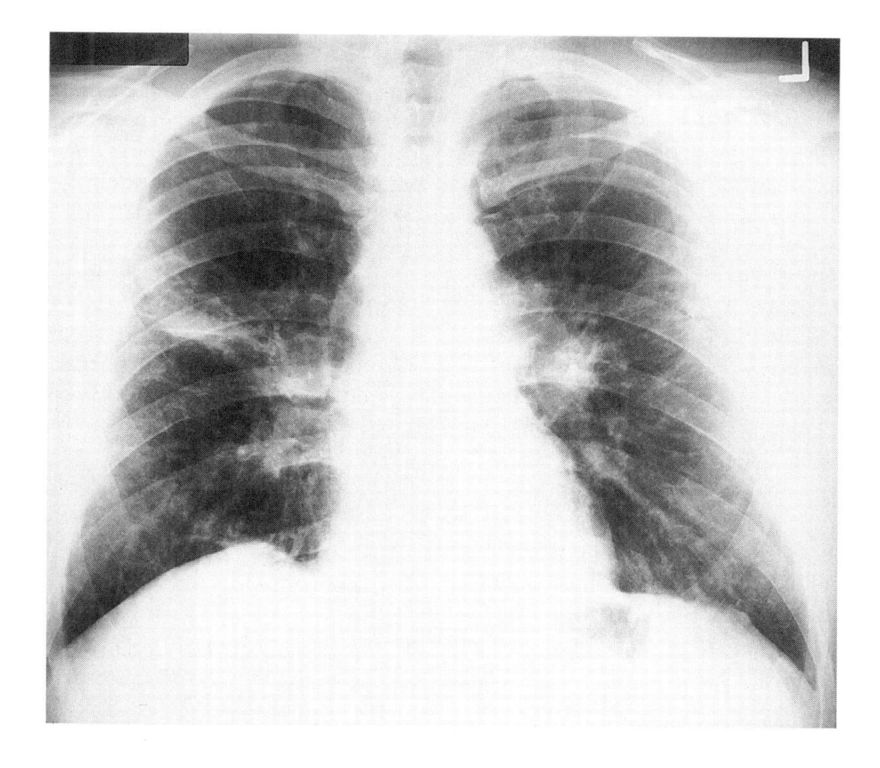

124. A 64-year-old woman is found to have a left-sided pleural effusion on chest x-ray. Analysis of the pleural fluid reveals a ratio of concentration of total protein in pleural fluid to serum of 0.38, a lactic dehydrogenase (LDH) level of 125 IU, and a ratio of LDH concentration in pleural fluid to serum of 0.46. Which of the following disorders is most likely in this patient?

a. Uremia
b. Congestive heart failure
c. Pulmonary embolism
d. Sarcoidosis
e. Systemic lupus erythematosus

125. A patient is found to have an unexpectedly high value for diffusing capacity. This finding is consistent with which of the following disorders?

a. Anemia
b. Cystic fibrosis
c. Emphysema
d. Intrapulmonary hemorrhage

126. Which of the following does not indicate a poor prognostic finding in asthma?

a. Silent chest
b. Hypercapnia
c. Thoracoabdominal paradox (paradoxical respiration)
d. Pulsus paradoxus of 5 mm Hg
e. Altered mental status

127. A 40-year-old man without a significant past medical history comes to the emergency room with a three-day history of fever and shaking chills, with a 15-minute episode of rigor, nonproductive cough, and anorexia, as well as the development of right-sided pleuritic chest pain and shortness of breath over the last 12 hours. A chest roentgenogram reveals a consolidated right middle lobe infiltrate, and a CBC shows an elevated neutrophil count with many band forms present. Which of the following statements regarding pneumonia in this patient is correct?

a. Sputum culture is more helpful than sputum Gram stain in choosing empiric antibiotic therapy
b. If the Gram stain revealed numerous gram-positive diplococci, numerous white blood cells, and few epithelial cells, *S. pneumoniae* would be the most likely diagnosis.
c. Although *Streptococcus pneumoniae* is the agent most likely to be the cause of this patient's pneumonia, this diagnosis would be very unlikely if blood cultures were negative
d. The absence of rigors would rule out a diagnosis of pneumococcal pneumonia
e. Penicillin is the drug of choice in all cases of pneumococcal pneumonia

Items 128–129

128. A 57-year-old man develops acute shortness of breath shortly after a 12-hour automobile ride. The patient consults his internist, and findings on physical examination are normal except for tachypnea and tachycardia. An electrocardiogram reveals sinus tachycardia but is otherwise normal. Which of the following is correct?

a. A definitive diagnosis can be made by history alone
b. The patient should be admitted to the hospital, and if there is no contraindication to anticoagulation, intravenous heparin should be started pending further testing
c. Normal findings upon examination of the lower extremities are extremely unusual in this clinical setting
d. Early treatment has little effect on overall mortality

129. The most important next step in the diagnosis of the patient above would be

a. Pulmonary angiogram
b. Ventilation-perfusion scan
c. D-dimer
d. Venous ultrasound

130. The most likely finding in a patient with acute pulmonary embolus is

a. Wheezing
b. Pleuritic chest pain
c. Tachypnea
d. Hemoptysis
e. Right-sided S_3 heart sound

131. A 65-year-old male with mild congestive heart failure is to receive total hip replacement. He has no other underlying diseases, no history of hypertension, recent surgery, or bleeding disorder. The best approach to prevention of pulmonary embolus in this patient is

a. Aspirin—75 mg per day
b. Aspirin—325 mg per day
c. Warfarin with INR of 2–3
d. Early ambulation

132. The hallmark of asthma that distinguishes it from other obstructive airway diseases is that in asthma

a. Hyperinflation is present on chest roentgenogram
b. Airway obstruction is reversible
c. Hypoxia occurs as a consequence of ventilation-perfusion mismatch
d. The FEV_1/FVC ratio is reduced
e. Exacerbation often occurs as a result of an upper respiratory tract infection

DIRECTIONS: Each group of questions below consists of lettered headings followed by a set of numbered items. For each numbered item select the **one** lettered heading with which it is most closely associated. Each lettered heading may be used once, more than once, or not at all.

Items 133–137

For each clinical picture below, select the arterial blood gas and pH values with which it is most likely to be associated

	pH	P_{O_2}	P_{CO_2}
a.	7.50	75	28
b.	7.15	78	92
c.	7.06	36	95
d.	7.06	108	13
e.	7.39	48	54

133. A 30-year-old obese female bus driver develops sudden pleuritic left-sided chest pain and dyspnea

134. A 60-year-old heavy smoker has severe chronic bronchitis and peripheral edema and cyanosis

135. A 22-year-old drug-addicted man is brought to the emergency room by friends who were unable to awaken him

136. A 62-year-old man who has chronic bronchitis and chest pain is given oxygen via mask in the ambulance en route to the hospital and becomes lethargic in the emergency room

137. A 20-year-old man with diabetes mellitus comes to the emergency room with diffuse abdominal pain, tachypnea, and a fever

Items 138–142

For each set of findings below, select the disease with which it is most likely to be associated.

a. Asthma
b. Rheumatoid arthritis
c. $Alpha_1$ antitrypsin deficiency
d. Cystic fibrosis
e. Sarcoidosis

138. Low levels of glucose in pleural effusions

139. Bronchiectasis and severe hemoptysis as frequent complications of clinical course

140. Presence of the mucoid strain of *Pseudomonas aeruginosa*

141. Development of severe liver disease that is usually associated with, but may be independent of, lung disease

142. Development of symptoms after ingestion of tartrazine yellow or aspirin

Items 143–146

For each pulmonary disorder below, select the disease with which it is most likely to be associated.

a. Scleroderma
b. Systemic lupus erythematosus (SLE)
c. Rheumatoid arthritis
d. Sjögren's syndrome

143. Pulmonary lymphoma

144. Pulmonary hypertension

145. Pulmonary nodules

146. Pleuritis and pericarditis

DIRECTIONS: Each item below contains a question or incomplete statement followed by suggested responses. Select the **one best** response to each question.

147. A 60-year-old male has had a chronic cough for over five years with clear sputum production. He smoked one pack of cigarettes per day for 20 years and continues to do so. X-ray of the chest shows hyperinflation without infiltrates. Arterial blood gases show a pH of 7.38, P_{CO_2} of 40 mm Hg, P_{O_2} of 65 mm Hg. Spirometry shows a FEV_1/FVC of 65%. The most important treatment modality for this patient would be

a. Oral corticosteroids
b. Home oxygen
c. Broad-spectrum antibiotics
d. Smoking cessation program

148. A 50-year-old male with emphysema and a chest x-ray that has shown apical blebs develops the sudden onset of shortness of breath and left-sided pleuritic chest pain. Pneumothorax is suspected. Physical examination findings that would confirm the diagnosis are

a. Localized wheezes at the left base
b. Hyperresonance of the left chest, decreased breath sounds
c. Increased tactile fremitus on the left side
d. Decreased breath sounds left side, trachea deviated to the left

149. A 30-year-old paraplegic male has a long history of urinary tract infection secondary to an indwelling Foley catheter. He develops fever and hypotension requiring hospitalization, fluid therapy, and intravenous antibiotics. He improves, but over one week becomes increasingly short of breath and tachypneic. He develops frothy sputum, diffuse rales, and diffuse alveolar infiltrates. There is no fever, jugular venous distention, S_3 gallop, or peripheral or sacral edema. The best approach to a definitive diagnosis in this patient would be

a. Blood cultures
b. CT scan of the chest
c. Pulmonary capillary wedge pressure
d. Ventilation-perfusion scan

PULMONARY DISEASE

Answers

108. The answer is b. *(Fauci, 14/e, pp 1953–1955.)* The clinical picture suggests hypertrophic osteoarthropathy. This process, the pathogenesis of which is unknown, is characterized by clubbing of digits, periosteal new bone formation, and arthritis. Hypertrophic osteoarthropathy is associated with intrathoracic malignancy, suppurative lung disease, and congenital heart problems. Treatment is directed at the underlying disease process. While x-rays may suggest osteomyelitis, the process is usually bilateral and easily distinguishable from osteomyelitis. The first step in evaluation of this patient is to obtain chest x-ray looking for lung infection and carcinoma.

109. The answer is b. *(Stobo, 23/e, pp 121–125.)* The diagnosis in this patient is suggested by the physical exam findings. The findings of poor excursion, flatness of percussion, and decreased fremitus on the right side are all consistent with a right-sided pleural effusion. A large right-sided effusion may shift the trachea to the left. A pneumothorax should result in hyperresonance of the affected side. Atelectasis on the right side would shift the trachea to the right. A consolidated pneumonia would characteristically result in increased fremitus and would not cause tracheal deviation.

110. The answer is b. *(Fauci, 14/e, p 1428.)* This 60-year-old woman has peripheral eosinophilia in association with pulmonary infiltrates. The differential diagnosis for eosinophilic pneumonia includes allergic bronchopulmonary aspergillosis, parasitic infections, drug reactions, and a category of idiopathic disease. Nitrofundantoin and sulfonamides are among the drugs most likely to cause eosinophilic pneumonia. Hypersensitivity pneumonitis may cause bilateral infiltrates, but does not, of itself, cause eosinophilia.

111. The answer is d. *(Fauci, 14/e, pp 994, 1438.)* Of the organisms listed, only anaerobic infection is likely to cause a necrotizing process. Type III pneumococci have been reported to cause cavitary disease, but this is unusual. The location of the infiltrate suggests aspiration, also making anaerobic infection most likely.

112–116. The answers are 112-b, 113-d, 114-a, 115-c, 116-e. *(Fauci, 14/e, pp 1472–1474.)* Congestive heart failure usually produces a right-sided pleural effusion. Of all the disease processes listed, it is the only one that usually results in a transudative effusion. Hence B (protein less than 3.0) is the best answer.

Tuberculosis causes an exudative lymphocytic effusion. Empyema may be defined by the very low pH value. It is an exudative effusion with a polymorphonuclear leukocyte predominance. Rheumatoid effusions are often exudative and may be lymphocytic, but they are best characterized by their very low glucose levels. Mesotheliomas produce a very bloody effusion.

117–120. The answers are 117-a, 118-b, 119-c, 120-d. *(Fauci, 14/e, pp 1009, 1291, 880.)* The patient, with fever, shaking chills, and a Gram stain showing gram-positive cocci in clusters, has staphylococcal aureus pneumonia. Chest x-ray A shows a necrotizing pneumonia characteristic of this infection. The patient with symptoms of shortness of breath and paroxysmal nocturnal dyspnea might have chest x-ray B, which shows signs of congestive heart failure including cardiomegaly, bilateral infiltrates, and cephalization. Chest x-ray C is best matched with the patient who has fever and night sweats. This x-ray shows characteristic changes of tuberculosis, including extensive apical and upper lobe scarring. The patient with long-standing hypertension shows chest x-ray evidence for left ventricular hypertrophy.

121. The answer is c. *(Fauci, 14/e, pp 2396, 326.)* Because the clinical signs of neurologic deterioration and a petechial rash have occurred in the setting of fracture and hypoxia, fat embolism is the most likely diagnosis. This process occurs when neutral fat is introduced into the venous circulation after bone trauma or fracture. The latent period is 12 to 36 hours, usually earlier than a pulmonary embolus would occur after trauma.

122. The answer is c. *(Fauci, 14/e, pp 1458–1459.)* When stupor and coma supervene in CO_2 retention, fatal arrhythmias, seizures, and death are likely to follow. Stopping oxygen is the worst course of action, as it will exacerbate life-threatening hypoxia. Intubation is the only good alternative. Bicarbonate plays no role in this acidosis, which is respiratory and caused by hypoventilation.

123. The answer is c. *(Fauci, 14/e, pp 1924–1925.)* Sarcoidosis is a systemic illness of unknown etiology. Many patients have respiratory symptoms, including cough and dyspnea. Hilar and peripheral lymphadenopathy is common, and 20 to 30% of patients have hepatomegaly. The chest x-ray shown shows symmetrical hilar lymphadenopathy. The diagnostic method of choice is transbronchial biopsy, which will show a mononuclear cell granulomatous inflammatory process. While liver and scalene-node biopsies are often positive, noncaseating granulomas are so frequent in these sites that they are not considered acceptable for primary diagnosis. ACE levels are elevated in two-thirds of patients, but false-positive values are common in other granulomatous disease processes.

124. The answer is b. *(Fauci, 13/e, pp 1472–1474.)* Classifying a pleural effusion as either a transudate or an exudate is useful in identifying the underlying disorder. Pleural fluid is exudative if it has any one of the following three properties: a ratio of concentration of total protein in pleural fluid to serum greater than 0.5, an absolute value of LDH greater than 200 IU, or a ratio of LDH concentration in pleural fluid to serum greater than 0.6. Causes of exudative effusions include malignancy, pulmonary embolism, pneumonia, tuberculosis, abdominal disease, collagen vascular diseases, uremia, Dressler's syndrome, and chylothorax. Exudative effusions may also be drug-induced. If none of the aforementioned properties are met, the effusion is a transudate. Differential diagnosis includes congestive heart failure, nephrotic syndrome, cirrhosis, Meigs' syndrome, and hydronephrosis.

125. The answer is d. *(Fauci, 14/e, pp 1410–1416.)* The carbon monoxide (CO) diffusing capacity provides an estimate of the rate at which oxygen moves by diffusion from alveolar gas to combine with hemoglobin in the red blood cells. It is interpreted as an index of the surface area engaged in alveolar-capillary diffusion. Measurement of diffusing capacity of the lung is done by having the person inspire a low concentration of carbon monoxide. The rate of uptake of the gas by the blood is calculated from the difference between the inspired and expired concentrations. The test can be performed during a single 10-second breath holding or during a minute of steady-state breathing. The diffusing capacity is defined as the amount of carbon monoxide transferred per minute per millimeter of mercury of driving pressure and correlates with oxygen transport from the alveolus into the capillaries. Primary parenchymal disorders, anemia, and removal of lung tissue decrease the diffusing capacity. Conversely, polycythemia, congestive heart failure, and intrapulmonary hemorrhage tend to increase the value for diffusing capacity.

126. The answer is d. *(Stobo, 23/e, p 143.)* It is extremely important to accurately determine the severity of an exacerbation of asthma, since the major cause of death from asthma is the underestimation of the severity of a particular episode by either the patient or the physician. Silent chest is a particularly ominous finding because the airway constriction is so great that airflow is insufficient to generate wheezing. Hypercapnia and thoracoabdominal paradox almost always are indicative of exhaustion and respiratory muscle failure or fatigue and generally need to be aggressively treated with mechanical ventilation. Altered mental status is frequently seen with severe hypoxia or hypercapnia, and ventilatory support is usually required. An increased pulsus paradoxus may also be a sign of severe asthma, as it increases with greater respiratory effort and generation of more negative intrathoracic pressures during inspiration. However, a pulsus paradoxus of up to 8 to 10 mm Hg is considered normal; thus, a value of 5 mm Hg would not be indicative of a severe episode of asthma.

127. The answer is b. *(Fauci, 14/e, pp 1437–1445.)* Pneumonia is a common disorder and is a major cause of death, particularly in hospitalized, elderly patients. Before choosing empiric therapy for presumed pneumonia, it is necessary to know the age of the patient, whether the infection is community-acquired or nosocomial, and whether there are any underlying debilitating illnesses. Community-acquired pneumonias in patients over the age of 35 are most likely due to *Streptococcus pneumoniae, Legionella* species (e.g., *pneumophila*), and *Haemophilus influenzae.* In the case outlined, the history is strongly consistent with pneumococcal pneumonia, manifest by a short prodrome, shaking chills with rigor, fever, chest pain, sparse sputum production associated with cough, and a consolidated lobar infiltrate on chest roentgenogram. The most reliable method of the diagnosis of pneumococcal pneumonia is seeing gram-positive diplococci on an adequate sputum (many white cells, few epithelial cells). Sputum culture is also important in the era of penicillin-resistant pneumococci, but is not helpful in initial diagnosis. Blood cultures are positive in only about 20% of patients, and when positive, are indicative of a more severe case. Although rigors may suggest pneumococcal bacteremia, the absence of rigors does not rule out the diagnosis. About 25% of pneumococci in the United States are partially or completely resistant to penicillin due to chromosomal mutations resulting in penicillin-binding protein changes. Penicillin is no longer the regimen of choice for pneumococcal pneumonia pending the results of sensitivity testing. The fluoroquinolones or ceftriaxone are widely used as initial therapy for pneumococcal pneumonia.

128. The answer is b. *(Fauci, 14/e, pp 1469–1472.)* The clinical situation described is characteristic of pulmonary embolic disease. Pulmonary emboli in greater than 80% of cases arise from thromboses in the deep-venous circulation (DVTs) of the lower extremities. DVTs often begin in the calf, where they rarely, if ever, cause clinically significant pulmonary embolic disease. However, thromboses that begin below the knee frequently "grow," or propagate, above the knee; clots that dislodge from above the knee cause clinically significant pulmonary emboli, which, if untreated, cause mortality exceeding 80%. Interestingly, only about 50% of patients with DVT of the lower extremities have clinical findings of swelling, warmth, erythema, pain, or "cords." As long as the superficial venous system, which has connections with the deep-venous system, remains patent, none of the classic clinical findings of DVT will occur, because blood will drain from the unobstructed superficial system. When a clot does dislodge from the deep-venous system and travels into the pulmonary vasculature, the most common clinical findings are tachypnea and tachycardia; chest pain is less likely and is more indicative of concomitant pulmonary infarction. The ABG is usually abnormal, and a high percentage of patients exhibit hypoxia, hypocapnia, alkalosis, and a widening of the alveolar-arterial gradient (P). The ECG is frequently abnormal in pulmonary embolic disease. The most common finding is sinus tachycardia, but atrial fibrillation, pseudoinfarction in the inferior leads, and right and left axis deviation are also occasionally seen. Initial treatment for suspected pulmonary embolic disease includes prompt hospitalization and institution of intravenous heparin, provided there are no contraindications to anticoagulation.

129. The answer is b. *(Fauci, 14/e, pp 1470–1471.)* Lung scanning is the principal imaging test for the diagnosis of pulmonary embolus. The diagnosis is very unlikely in patients with normal or near-normal scans. The diagnosis is highly likely in patients with high probability scans. In patients with a high clinical index of suspicion for pulmonary embolus but low-probability scan, the diagnosis becomes more difficult, and pulmonary angiography may be indicated. About two-thirds of patients with pulmonary embolus have evidence of deep-venous disease by venous ultrasound. Therefore, pulmonary embolus cannot be excluded by a normal study. The quantitative D-dimer enzyme-linked immunoabsorbent assay is positive in 90% of patients with pulmonary embolus in some studies. It has been used to rule out pulmonary embolus in a patient with a low- or intermediate-probability scan.

130. The answer is c. *(Stein, 5/e, pp 500–501.)* While all of these signs and symptoms can occur in acute pulmonary embolus, tachypnea is by far the most common. Pleuritic chest occurs in about half of patients and is less common in the elderly and those with underlying heart disease. Hemoptysis and wheezing occur in less than half of patients. A right-sided S_3 sound is associated with large emboli that result in acute pulmonary hypertension.

131. The answer is c. *(Stein, 5/e, p 504.)* Warfarin is the principal agent recommended for the prophylaxis of acute pulmonary embolus in patients who receive total hip replacement. Warfarin is started preoperatively, and the daily dose is adjusted to maintain an international normalized ratio (INR) of 2 to 3. The value of aspirin in this setting is unclear. Early ambulation and elastic stockings are also important in preventing thromboembolism, but are not adequate in themselves in this high-risk situation.

132. The answer is b. *(Fauci, 14/e, p 1423.)* Asthma is an incompletely understood inflammatory process that involves the lower airways and results in bronchoconstriction and excess production of mucus, which in turn lead to increased airway resistance and occasionally respiratory failure and death. During acute exacerbations of asthma, and in other obstructive lung diseases such as chronic obstructive pulmonary disease, hyperinflation may be present on chest roentgenogram, hypoxia is common and usually a result of ventilation-perfusion mismatch, the FEV_1/FVC is reduced, and exacerbations are frequently precipitated by upper airway infections. Only in asthma is the airway obstruction reversible.

133–137. The answers are 133-a, 134-e, 135-c, 136-b, 137-d. *(Stobo, 23/e, pp 121–125, 162–176, 155–158.)* The blood-gas values associated with pulmonary embolism may vary tremendously. The most consistent finding is acute respiratory alkalosis. It is important to note that hypoxemia, although frequently found, need not be present.

In severe chronic lung disease, the presence of hypercapnia leads to a compensatory increase in serum bicarbonate. Thus, significant hypercapnia may be present with an arterial pH close to normal, but will never be completely corrected.

Acute respiratory acidosis may occur secondary to respiratory depression after drug overdose. Hypoventilation is associated with hypoxia, hypercapnia, and severe, uncompensated acidosis. In the presence of longstanding lung disease, respiration may become regulated in hypoxia rather than by altered carbon dioxide tension and arterial pH, as in normal people. Thus, the unmonitored administration of oxygen may lead to respiratory suppression, as in the patient described in the question, that results in acute and chronic respiratory acidosis. Young patients with type 1 diabetes mellitus may present with rapid onset of diabetic ketoacidosis (DKA), usually secondary to a systemic infection. These patients usually are maximally ventilating, as indicated by a very low arterial P_{CO_2}; however, they remain acidotic secondary to the severe metabolic ketoacidosis associated with this process. In general, these patients are not hypoxic unless the underlying infection is pneumonia.

138–142. The answers are 138-b, 139-d, 140-d, 141-c, 142-a. *(Fauci, 14/e, pp 1448–1451, 1884, 1473.)* Asthma is predominantly an inflammatory lower airway process. Frequent triggers of airway inflammation, and thus asthma, include infection, inhaled allergens, and processes that cool or dry the airways, such as exercise and exposure to cold weather. In addition, certain chemicals, such as aspirin (but not sodium or magnesium salicylate) and tartrazine yellow, have been implicated in the development of bronchospasm in certain patients.

Pleural effusions are not unusual in patients with rheumatoid arthritis. A history of pleurodynia that would suggest an antecedent inflammatory pleuritis is not always obtained, but characteristically, the pleural fluid, which is sterile, will contain a high level of lactic dehydrogenase and a low glucose concentration. Other pulmonary phenomena associated with rheumatoid arthritis include diffuse interstitial fibrosis and the occurrence of individual or clustered nodules in the lung parenchyma.

The fatality rate for patients with cystic fibrosis is lower today than in previous years; the average life span of patients afflicted with this disease has been significantly increasing. Chronic lung infections, however, are almost universal. The most common and difficult to treat of such infections is caused by the mucoid strain of *Pseudomonas aeruginosa*. Chronic coughing is one of the major and most distressing problems of patients with cystic fibrosis. Liver disease, particularly biliary cirrhosis, may develop in these patients. Common pulmonary complications include bronchiectasis, severe hemoptysis, and allergic bronchopulmonary aspergillosis. The incidence of liver disease associated with a deficiency of $alpha_1$ antitrypsin is very high. Patients with liver disease secondary to $alpha_1$ antitrypsin deficiency usually, but not always, have accompanying panacinar emphysema.

Sarcoidosis is a nonspecific granulomatous disease of unknown etiology. Blacks and Mediterranean peoples appear to be predisposed. The most commonly involved organs—after the lungs—are liver, eye, spleen, skin, and kidney. The most characteristic presentation is a patient with a nonproductive cough with bilateral hilar adenopathy on chest x-ray. Treatment with prednisone is usually reserved for patients with diminishing pulmonary function, evidenced by reduced diffusing capacity or reduced lung volumes; 70 to 80% of untreated, stable patients will spontaneously remit.

143–146. The answers are 143-d, 144-a, 145-c, 146-b. *(Fauci, 14/e, pp 1903, 1912–1916, 1877.)* Connective tissue disorders frequently have pulmonary manifestations. There may be significant overlap in the pulmonary involvement seen among the connective tissue disorders. In addition, the spectrum of disease seen in any of these disorders may make it hard to accurately classify a particular patient. SLE, perhaps the most common of these disorders, can exhibit many different pulmonary manifestations. Pleuritis and pericarditis are the most common. Other types of pulmonary involvement include vasculitis, interstitial fibrosis, pulmonary hemorrhage, elevation of the diaphragm and loss of lung volume ("vanishing lung syndrome"), and, rarely, pulmonary hypertension.

Rheumatoid arthritis, another common disorder, can cause pleuritis and pleural effusion as in SLE; however, pericarditis is rare. Pulmonary nodules are seen frequently in this disorder, and they are usually asymptomatic.

In scleroderma, interstitial fibrosis is the most common pulmonary complication. Pulmonary hypertension, although relatively uncommon, is more likely to occur in scleroderma than in other connective tissue disorders.

The most common clinical feature of Sjögren's syndrome is keratoconjunctivitis sicca, in which patients have diminished salivary gland production and present with dry mouth and eyes. The most common pulmonary manifestation of this disorder is dry cough, although airway obstruction may be seen in about 10% of cases. An interesting association with this disorder is lymphoma, as patients with Sjögren's syndrome are at a fortyfold greater risk of developing lymphoma compared with the general population. Occasionally, these lymphomas will primarily involve the lung.

147. The answer is d. *(Stobo, 23/e, pp 138–139.)* This patient's chronic cough, hyperinflated lung fields, abnormal pulmonary function tests, and smoking history are all consistent with chronic bronchitis. A smoking cessation program can decrease the rate of lung deterioration and is successful in as many as 40% of patients, particularly when the physician gives a strong antismoking message and uses both counseling and nicotine replacement. Continuous low-flow oxygen becomes beneficial when arterial oxygen concentration falls below 55 mm Hg. Antibiotics are indicated only for acute exacerbations of chronic lung disease, which might present with fever, change in color of sputum, and increasing shortness of breath. Oral corticosteroids are helpful in some patients, but are reserved for those who have failed inhaled bronchodilator treatments.

148. The answer is b. *(Stein, 5/e, pp 510–511.)* The most characteristic findings of a pneumothorax are hyperresonance and decreased breath sounds. A tension pneumothorax may displace the mediastinum to the unaffected side. Tactile fremitus would be decreased in the patient with a pneumothorax, but would be increased in conditions in which consolidation of the lung had developed.

149. The answer is c. Sepsis is the most important single cause of adult respiratory distress syndrome. Early in the course of ARDS, patients may appear stable without respiratory symptoms. Tachypnea, hypoxemia, and diffuse infiltrates gradually develop. It may be difficult to distinguish the process from cardiogenic pulmonary edema, especially in patients who have been given large quantities of fluid. This young patient with no evidence of volume overload would be strongly suspected of having ARDS. The pulmonary capillary wedge pressure would be normal or low in ARDS, but elevated in left ventricular failure. ARDS is a complication of sepsis, but blood cultures may or may not be positive. Neither CT of the chest nor ventilation-perfusion scan would be specific enough to help in diagnosis of ARDS.

CARDIOLOGY

DIRECTIONS: Each item below contains a question or incomplete statement followed by suggested responses. Select the **one best** response to each question.

150. Your 60-year-old male patient, followed for chronic stable angina on aspirin, nitrates, and a beta blocker, presents to the ER with history of two to three episodes of more severe and long-lasting anginal chest pain each day over the past three days. His ECG and cardiac enzymes are normal. The best course of action of the following is to

a. Admit the patient and begin intravenous digoxin
b. Admit the patient and begin intravenous heparin
c. Admit the patient and give prophylactic thrombolytic therapy
d. Admit the patient for observation with no change in medication
e. Discharge the patient from the ER with increases in nitrates and beta blockers

151. A 60-year-old white female presents with epigastric pain, nausea and vomiting, heart rate of 50, and transient second-degree AV block Mobitz type II on ER cardiac monitor. Blood pressure is 130/80. The coronary artery most likely to be involved in this process is the

a. Right coronary artery
b. Left main
c. Left anterior descending
d. Circumflex

152. The classic presentation of acute myocardial infarction (MI) involves heavy or crushing substernal chest pain. The type of patient most likely to present with painless, or *silent,* MI is the

a. Advanced coronary artery disease patient with unstable angina
b. Elderly diabetic
c. Premenopausal female
d. Inferior MI patient
e. MI patient with PVCs

153. A 75-year-old African American female was admitted with acute myocardial infarction and congestive heart failure, then had an episode of ventricular tachycardia. She is prescribed multiple medications and soon develops confusion and slurred speech. The most likely cause of this confusion is

a. Captopril
b. Digoxin
c. Furosemide
d. Lidocaine
e. Nitroglycerin

154. Two weeks after hospital discharge for documented myocardial infarction, a 65-year-old returns to your office very concerned about low-grade fever and pleuritic chest pain. There is no associated shortness of breath. Lungs are clear to auscultation and heart exam is free of significant murmurs, gallops, or rubs. ECG is unchanged from the last one in the hospital. The most effective therapy would likely be

a. Antibiotics
b. Anticoagulation with warfarin (Coumadin)
c. An anti-inflammatory agent
d. An increase in antianginal medication
e. An antianxiety agent

155. A 72-year-old male presents to the ER with history of paroxysmal nocturnal dyspnea and night cough along with physical exam findings of positive hepatojugular reflux, rales, and S_3 gallop. Which of the following is not a major criteria for congestive heart failure according to Framingham criteria?

a. Paroxysmal nocturnal dyspnea
b. Night cough
c. Positive hepatojugular reflux
d. Rales
e. S_3 gallop

156. A precipitating cause of high-output cardiac failure, which might present as described in the preceding question, is

a. Alcoholic cardiomyopathy
b. Hypertension
c. Myocardial infarction
d. Multiple PVCs
e. Thyrotoxicosis

157. Your 55-year-old patient presents back to you with history of having recently had a myocardial infarction with a five-day hospital stay while away on a business trip. He reports being told he had mild congestive heart failure then, but is asymptomatic now with normal physical exam. You would recommend which of the following medications:

a. An ACE inhibitor
b. Digoxin
c. Furosemide (Lasix)
d. Hydralazine
e. Nitrates

158. A 26-year-old-female is referred to you from an OB-GYN colleague due to the onset of extreme fatigue and dyspnea on exertion three months after her second vaginal delivery. By history, physical, and adjunctive tests, including echocardiogram, you make the diagnosis of postpartum cardiomyopathy. Which of the following is correct?

a. Postpartum cardiomyopathy may occur unexpectedly years after pregnancy and delivery
b. About half of all patients will recover completely
c. Since the condition is idiosyncratic, future pregnancy may be entered into with no greater than average risk
d. The postpartum state will require a different therapeutic approach than typical dilated cardiomyopathies

159. Yesterday you admitted a 55-year-old white male to the hospital due to chest pain and ruled out MI. He tends to be anxious about his health. On admission, his lungs were clear, and his heart revealed a grade I/VI early systolic murmur over the precordium; cardiac enzymes were normal, and ECG showed right bundle branch block. The idea of performing a routine Bruce protocol treadmill exercise test (stress test) to further assess coronary artery disease was considered, but rejected primarily due to which of the following?

a. Anticipated difficulty with the patient's anxiety (i.e., he might falsely claim chest pain during the test)
b. Pulmonary embolus suspected as the primary diagnosis
c. Concern about the presence of aortic stenosis, a contraindication to stress testing
d. The presence of RBBB, with this baseline ECG change obscuring typical diagnostic ST-T changes
e. Concern that this represents the onset of unstable angina with unacceptable risk of MI with stress testing

160. A seventy-five-year-old patient presents to the ER after a sudden syncopal episode. He is again alert and in retrospect describes occasional substernal chest pressure and shortness of breath on exertion. His lungs have a few bibasilar rales and his blood pressure is 110/80. On cardiac auscultation, the classic finding you expect to hear is

a. A harsh systolic crescendo-decrescendo murmur heard best at the upper right sternal border
b. A diastolic decrescendo murmur heard at the mid-left sternal border
c. A holosystolic murmur heard best at the apex
d. A mid-systolic click

161. A seventy-two-year-old male comes to the office with intermittent symptoms of dyspnea on exertion, palpitations, and cough, occasionally productive of blood. On cardiac auscultation, a low-pitched diastolic rumbling murmur is faintly heard toward the apex. The origin of the patient's problem probably relates to

a. Rheumatic fever as a youth
b. Long-standing hypertension
c. Silent MI within the past year
d. Congenital

162. You are helping with school sports physicals and see a 13-year-old boy who has had some trouble keeping up with his peers. He has a cardiac murmur, which you correctly diagnose as a ventricular septal defect based on the following auscultatory finding:

a. A systolic crescendo-decrescendo murmur heard best at the upper right sternal border with radiation to the carotids; the murmur is augmented with transient exercise
b. A systolic murmur at the pulmonic area and a diastolic rumble along the left sternal border
c. A holosystolic murmur at the mid-left sternal border
d. A diastolic decrescendo murmur at the mid-left sternal border
e. A continuous murmur through systole and diastole at the upper left sternal border

Items 163–164

163. A 40-year-old male presents to the office with history of palpitations that last for a few seconds and occur two or three times a week. There are no other symptoms. ECG shows a rare single unifocal premature ventricular contraction (PVC). The most likely cause of this finding is

a. Underlying coronary artery disease
b. Valvular heart disease
c. Hypertension
d. Apathetic hyperthyroidism
e. Idiopathic or unknown

164. Subsequent 24-hour Holter monitoring in the preceding patient confirms occasional single unifocal PVCs plus occasional premature atrial contractions (PACs). The most likely antiarrhythmic management in this case would be

a. Anxiolytics
b. Beta-blocker therapy
c. Digoxin
d. Quinidine
e. Observation, no medication

165. An active 78-year-old female has been followed for hypertension but presents with new onset of mild left hemiparesis and the finding of atrial fibrillation on ECG. She had been in sinus rhythm six months earlier. Optimal treatment by hospital discharge includes antihypertensives plus

a. Close observation
b. Permanent pacemaker
c. Aspirin
d. Warfarin (Coumadin)
e. Subcutaneous heparin

Items 166–167

166. A 36-year-old white female nurse comes to the ER due to a sensation of fast heart rate, slight dizziness, and vague chest fullness. The following rhythm strip is obtained which shows

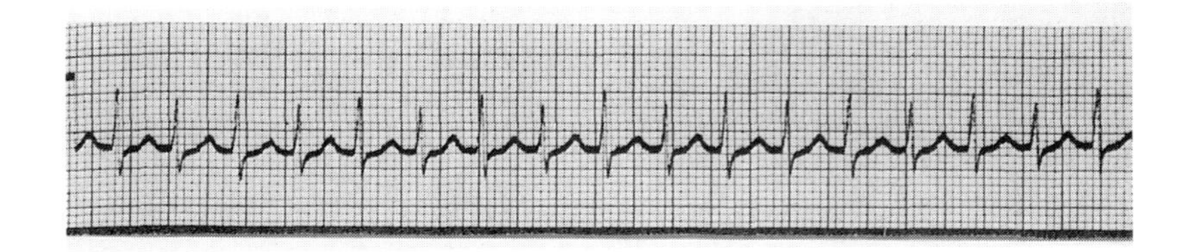

a. Atrial fibrillation
b. Atrial flutter
c. Supraventricular tachycardia
d. Ventricular tachycardia

167. The initial therapy of choice in this stable patient is

a. Adenosine 6 mg rapid IV bolus
b. Verapamil 2.5 to 5 mg IV over 1 to 2 minutes
c. Diltiazem 0.25 mg/kg IV over 2 minutes
d. Digoxin 0.5 mg IV slowly
e. Lidocaine 1.5 mg/kg IV bolus
f. Electrical cardioversion at 50 joules

168. A 65-year-old man with diabetes, on an oral hypoglycemic, presents to the ER with a sports-related right shoulder injury. His heart rate was noted to be irregular and the following ECG obtained. The best immediate therapy is

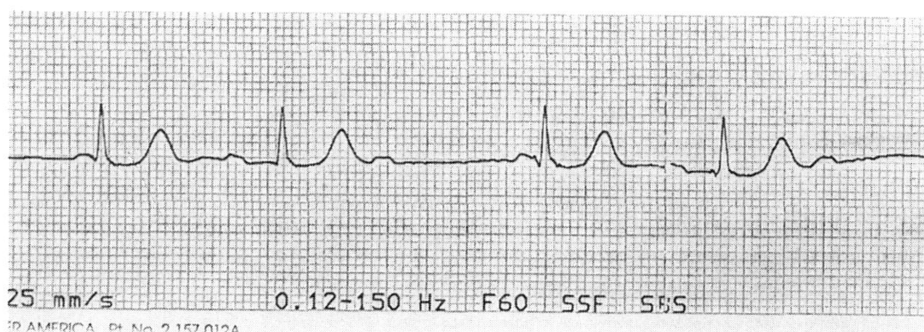

a. Atropine
b. Isoproterenol
c. Pacemaker
d. Electrical cardioversion
e. Digoxin
f. Diltiazem
g. Observation

169. While at the grocery store, you see an elderly lady slump to the floor. Going to her aid, your first step in Adult Basic Life Support (CPR) should be the following:

a. Check for a carotid pulse
b. Assess breathing
c. Establish an airway
d. Determine the individual's responsiveness
e. Institute chest compression

170. In the ICU, a patient suddenly becomes unresponsive, pulseless, and hypotensive, with cardiac monitor indicating ventricular tachycardia. The crash cart is immediately available. The first therapeutic step should be

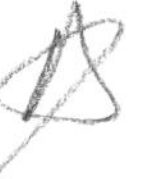

a. A precordial thump
b. Lidocaine 1.5 mg/kg IV push
c. Epinephrine 1 mg IV push
d. Defibrillation with 200 joules
e. Defibrillation with 360 joules

171. A 55-year-old African American female presents to the ER with lethargy and finding of blood pressure 250/150. Her family members indicate that she was complaining of severe headache and visual disturbance earlier in the day. They report a past history of asthma but no known kidney disease. The best approach is

a. IV labetalol therapy
b. Continuous infusion nitroprusside
c. Clonidine by mouth to lower blood pressure slowly but surely
d. Nifedipine sublingually to lower blood pressure rapidly and remove patient from danger
e. Further history about recent home antihypertensives before deciding current therapy

Items 172–173

An 18-year-old male complains of fever and transient pain in both knees and elbows. The right knee was red and swollen for one day the week prior to presentation. On physical exam, the patient has a low-grade fever but appears generally well. There is an aortic diastolic murmur heard at the base of the heart. A nodule is palpated over the extensor tendon of the hand. There are pink erythematous lesions over the abdomen, some with central clearing. The following laboratory values are obtained:

Hct: 42
WBC: 12,000/mm^3
20% polymorphonuclear leukocytes
80% lymphocytes
ESR: 60 mm/h

The patient's ECG is shown on the facing page.

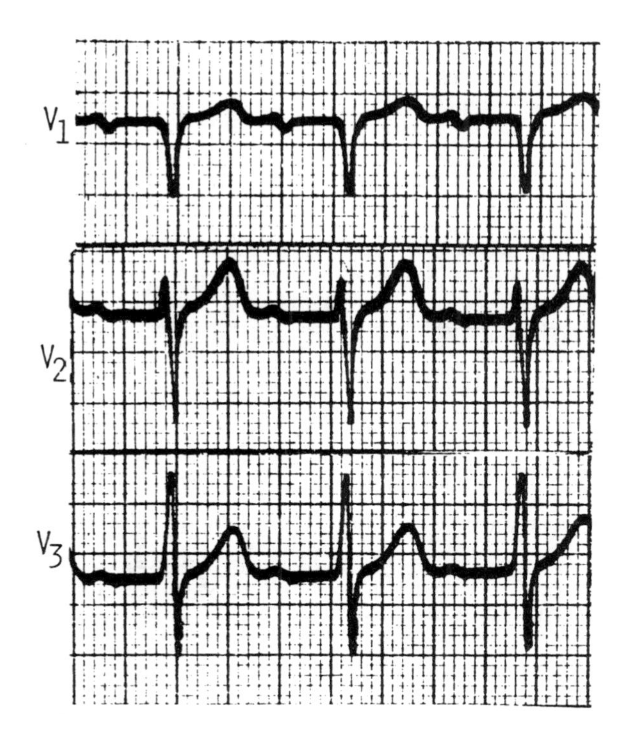

172. Which of the following tests is most critical to diagnosis?

a. Blood cultures
b. Antistreptolysin O antibody
c. Echocardiogram
d. Antinuclear antibodies
e. Creatinine phosphokinase

173. Based on the data available, the best approach to therapy would be

a. Ceftriaxone
b. Corticosteroids plus penicillin
c. Acetaminophen
d. Penicillin plus streptomycin
e. Ketoconazole

174. A patient has been in the cardiac care unit with an acute anterior myocardial infarction. He develops the abnormal rhythm shown below. You would

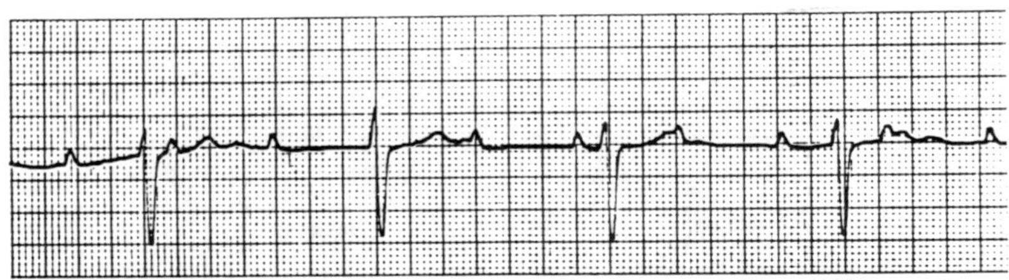

(Reproduced with permission, from Davis D. How to Quickly and Accurately Master EKG Interpre2 tation. Philadelphia, PA, Lippincott, 1985.)

a. Give digoxin
b. Consult for pacemaker
c. Perform cardioversion
d. Obtain digoxin level
e. Give lidocaine

175. A 48-year-old male with a history of hypercholesterolemia presents to the ER after one hour of substernal chest pain, nausea, and sweating. His ECG is shown at right. There is no history of hypertension, stroke, or any other serious illness. Which of the following therapies would be inappropriate?

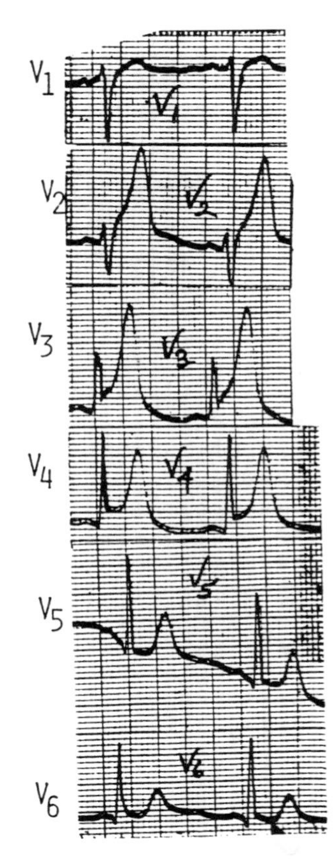

a. Aspirin
b. Beta blocker
c. Morphine
d. Digoxin
e. Nitroglycerin
f. Thrombolytic agent

176. A 55-year-old obese woman develops pressure-like substernal chest pain of one-hour duration. Her ECG is shown below. The most likely diagnosis is

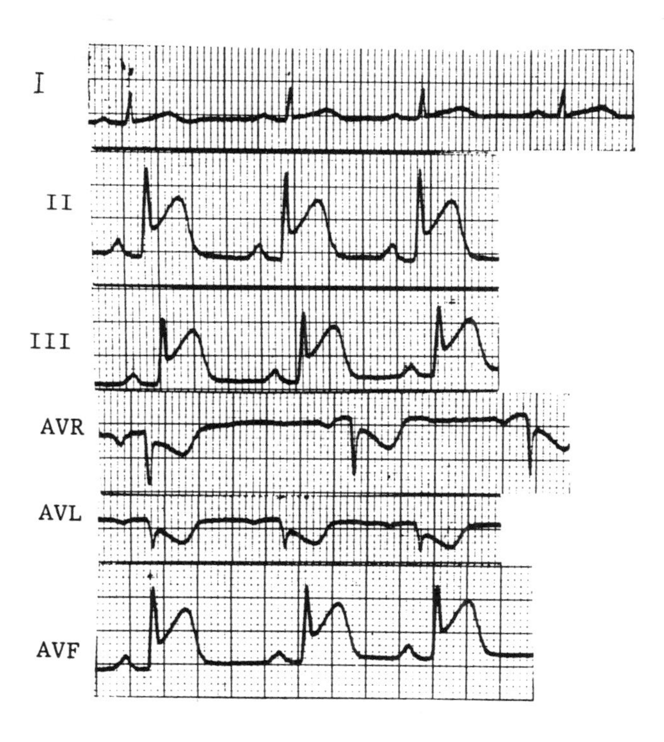

a. Costochondritis
b. Acute anterior myocardial infarction
c. Acute inferior myocardial infarction
d. Pericarditis
e. Esophageal reflux
f. Cholecystitis

177. A 50-year-old construction worker continues to have an elevated blood pressure of 160/95 even after a third agent is added to the hypertension regimen. Physical exam is normal, electrolytes are normal, and the patient is taking no over-the-counter medications. The next helpful step for this patient is to

a. Check pill count
b. Evaluate for Cushing's syndrome
c. Check chest x-ray for coarctation of aorta
d. Obtain renal angiogram

178. A 60-year-old female cigarette smoker complains of fatigue and dyspnea. The most specific evidence for congestive heart failure in this patient would be

a. Ankle edema
b. Wheezes
c. S_3 gallop
d. Weight gain

Items 179–180

A 35-year-old male complains of substernal chest pain, aggravated by inspiration and relieved by sitting up. The patient has had a history of tuberculosis. Chest x-ray shows an enlarged cardiac silhouette. Lung fields are clear.

179. The next step in evaluation would be

a. Right lateral decubitus film
b. Cardiac catheterization
c. Echocardiogram
d. Serial ECGs
e. Thallium stress test

180. The patient develops jugular venous distention. There is an inward movement of the jugular pulse synchronous with the pulse of the carotid artery. The ECG shows electrical alternans. The most likely additional finding would be

a. Basilar rales halfway up both posterior lung fields
b. S_3 gallop
c. Pulsus paradoxus
d. Strong apical beat

181. A 43-year-old woman with a one-year history of episodic leg edema and dyspnea is noted to have clubbing of the fingers. Her ECG is shown below. The correct diagnosis is

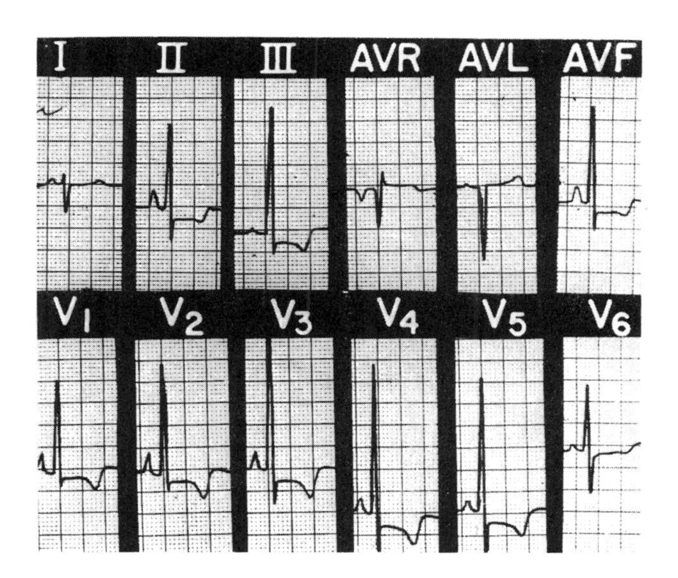

a. Inferior wall myocardial infarction
b. Right bundle branch block
c. Acute pericarditis
d. Wolff-Parkinson-White syndrome
e. Cor pulmonale

182. Which of the following statements correctly describes the most common primary cardiac tumor?

a. The majority are located in the left ventricle
b. It occurs more commonly in men than in women
c. Clinical presentation usually mimics mitral valve disease
d. It is histologically malignant
e. Peak incidence occurs in the second decade of life

183. The rhythm strip displayed below demonstrates

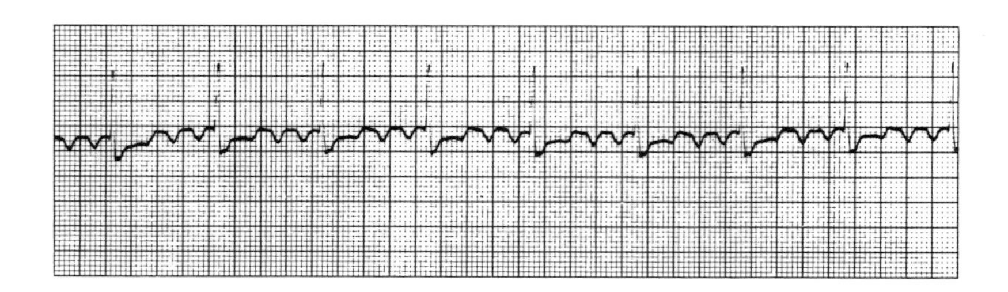

a. Normal sinus rhythm
b. Junctional rhythm
c. Atrial flutter with 4:1 atrioventricular block
d. Paroxysmal atrial tachycardia with 2:1 atrioventricular block
e. Complete heart block with 2:1 atrioventricular block

184. In a 30-year-old asymptomatic female with newly diagnosed mitral valve prolapse, which of the following is true?

a. Echocardiography demonstrates displacement of one or both mitral valve leaflets posteriorly into the left atrium during systole
b. Migration of the systolic click and systolic murmur toward the first heart sound will occur during squatting
c. Prophylactic beta-blocker therapy is indicated
d. Significant mitral regurgitation is likely to occur (>50% chance) sometime in her life
e. Restriction of exercise is advised to reduce the risk of sudden cardiac death

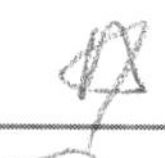

185. Which of the following cardiac conditions creates the lowest risk for development of infective endocarditis?

a. Coarctation of the aorta
b. Ventricular septal defect
c. Atrial septal defect
d. Prosthetic heart valve
e. Patent ductus arteriosus

186. An 80-year-old with past history of myocardial infarction is found to have left bundle branch block on ECG. He is asymptomatic with blood pressure 130/80, lungs clear to auscultation, and no leg edema. On cardiac auscultation the most likely finding is

a. Fixed (wide) split S_2
b. Paradoxically (reversed) split S_2
c. S_3
d. S_4
e. Opening snap
f. Mid-systolic click

DIRECTIONS: Each group of questions below consists of lettered headings followed by a set of numbered items. For each numbered item select the lettered heading with which it is most closely associated. Each lettered heading may be used once, more than once, or not at all. **Choose exactly the number of options indicated following each item.**

Items 187–189

Match the physical findings with the most likely valvular or related heart disease.

a. Mitral stenosis
b. Tricuspid regurgitation
c. Mitral regurgitation
d. Aortic regurgitation
e. Aortic stenosis
f. Hypertrophic cardiomyopathy

187. High-pitched, blowing, decrescendo, diastolic murmur. Widened arterial pulse pressure. **(SELECT ONE DISORDER)**

188. Holosystolic murmur at left sternal border; increased murmur on inspiration; prominent *v* wave in neck. **(SELECT ONE DISORDER)**

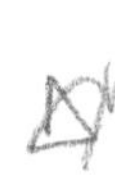

189. Crescendo-decrescendo systolic murmur beginning well after S_1, heard best at the lower left sternal border; rapidly rising carotid arterial pulse. **(SELECT ONE DISORDER)**

Items 190–194

For each clinical setting, choose the best next step in management from the following choices:

a. Digoxin
b. Propranolol
c. Calcium channel blocker
d. Atropine
e. Heparin
f. Lidocaine
g. Isoproterenol
h. Angiotensin converting enzyme inhibitor
i. Observation

190. Two-hour history of chest pain; acute ST-segment elevation in leads 2, 3, and AVF: sinus bradycardia at rate of 40 with hypotension. **(SELECT ONE STEP)**

191. Sudden onset of chest pain at night; ST-segment elevations in precordial leads. **(SELECT ONE STEP)**

192. Long-standing congestive heart failure (CHF); agent to act on arterial and venous beds and improve mortality. **(SELECT ONE STEP)**

193. Development of accelerated idioventricular rhythm with rate of 80. **(SELECT ONE STEP)**

194. Shortness of breath, palpitations, bifid apical beat, and increased intensity of systolic murmur on Valsalva maneuver. **(SELECT ONE STEP)**

Items 195–198

Match each situation with the correct description of splitting of the second heart sound.

a. Second heart sound splits into two components during inspiration
b. Second heart sound splits on expiration, with inspiratory fusion
c. Second sound is widely split; interval between sounds is fixed and unrelated to respiration
d. Second heart sound becomes more widely split on inspiration than is usual
e. No splitting of second heart sound in inspiration or expiration

195. Normal patient **(SELECT ONE SOUND)**

196. Severe aortic stenosis **(SELECT ONE SOUND)**

197. Right bundle branch block **(SELECT ONE SOUND)**

198. Atrial septal defect **(SELECT ONE SOUND)**

Items 199–204

Match the cardiac and/or antihypertensive agents below with associated side effects.

a. Increased triglyceride levels
b. Volume retention
c. Lupus-like syndrome
d. Cough
e. Gynecomastia
f. Rebound hypertension
g. First-dose syncope
h. Cyanide toxicity
i. Urinary retention

199. Captopril **(SELECT ONE EFFECT)**

200. Hydralazine **(SELECT ONE EFFECT)**

201. Propranolol **(SELECT ONE EFFECT)**

202. Minoxidil **(SELECT ONE EFFECT)**

203. Spironolactone **(SELECT ONE EFFECT)**

204. Terazosin **(SELECT ONE EFFECT)**

Items 205–208

For each electrolyte abnormality below, select the electrocardiographic finding with which it is most commonly associated.

a. No known electrocardiographic abnormalities
b. Prolonged QT interval
c. Short QT interval
d. Widened QRS complex
e. Prominent U waves

205. Hypokalemia **(SELECT ONE ECG FINDING)**

206. Hyperkalemia **(SELECT ONE ECG FINDING)**

207. Hypocalcemia **(SELECT ONE ECG FINDING)**

208. Hyponatremia **(SELECT ONE ECG FINDING)**

CARDIOLOGY

Answers

150. The answer is b. *(Alexander, 9/e, pp 1324–1327.)* This patient presents with unstable angina, a change from the previous chronic stable state in that chest pain has become more frequent and more severe. Intravenous heparin is indicated. There is no role for digoxin. Thrombolytic therapy is reserved for the treatment of ECG-documented myocardial infarction.

151. The answer is a. *(Alexander, 9/e, pp 52–55.)* The right coronary artery supplies most of the inferior myocardium and supplies the AV node in 80 to 90% of patients. Thus occlusion of this artery can cause ischemia of the AV node with AV block or bradycardia, as well as symptoms of an inferior MI as seen in this patient. AV block can occur with anterior MI related to LAD occlusion, but this generally implies a greater area of myocardial involvement and hemodynamic instability.

152. The answer is b. *(Fauci, 14/e, p 1353.)* The history of chest pain is the most common presenting complaint in myocardial infarction. However, 15 to 20% of infarctions may be painless, with the greatest incidence in diabetics and the elderly. Dyspnea or weakness may initially predominate in these patients. Diabetics are likely to have abnormal or absent pain response to myocardial ischemia due to generalized autonomic nervous system dysfunction.

153. The answer is d. *(Alexander, 9/e, p 975.)* While the clinical picture itself could lead to these neurological symptoms, the only cardiovascular medication on this list likely to do so is lidocaine. Lidocaine is particularly likely to cause confusion in the elderly patient, for whom a lower dose of the drug should generally be given.

154. The answer is c. *(Fauci, 14/e, pp 1363–1364.)* The history and physical are consistent with postmyocardial infarction syndrome (Dressler's syndrome) rather than infection, pulmonary embolus, angina, or anxiety. This syndrome represents an autoimmune pleuritis, pneumonitis, or pericarditis characterized by fever and pleuritic chest pain, with onset days to six weeks post-MI. Therefore the most effective therapy is a nonsteroidal anti-inflammatory drug.

155. The answer is b. *(Fauci, 14/e, pp 1290–1291.)* Night cough may occur in association with heart failure but is considered one of the minor criteria for congestive heart failure. Night cough is also a common symptom in asthma. Major criteria for the diagnosis of congestive heart failure include paroxysmal nocturnal dyspnea, hepatojugular reflux, rales, S_3 gallop, neck vein distention, cardiomegaly, acute pulmonary edema, and increased venous pressure. The Framingham criteria include eight major and seven minor criteria. To establish a clinical diagnosis of congestive heart failure, at least one major and two minor criteria are required.

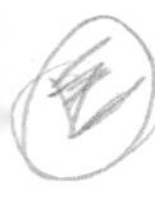

156. The answer is e. *(Fauci, 14/e, pp 1287–1288.)* Thyrotoxicosis is an important cause of high-output congestive heart failure. Other possibilities in the high-output category are infection, anemia, pregnancy, AV fistulas, beriberi, and Paget's disease. In evaluating patients with heart failure it is important to identify not only underlying causes of heart disease but also precipitating factors that place an additional load on an already burdened myocardium.

157. The answer is a. *(Fauci, 14/e, p 1291.)* The administration of an angiotensin converting enzyme inhibitor has been shown to retard the development of heart failure and should be begun as early as possible in patients with cardiac dilatation or hypertrophy, even in asymptomatic patients. As symptoms develop, restriction of activity and dietary sodium should be instituted.

158. The answer is b. *(Alexander, 9/e, p 2049.)* Postpartum (or peripartum) cardiomyopathy may occur during the last trimester of pregnancy or within six months of delivery. About half of patients will recover completely, with most of the rest improving. However, current advice is to avoid future pregnancies due to risk of recurrence.

159. The answer is d. *(Alexander, 9/e, p 522.)* ST-segment depression is the most common manifestation of exercise-induced myocardial ischemia.

This type of change is difficult to assess in the presence of any bundle branch block in which the ST segment is already abnormal. In this case, an exercise test with radionuclide imaging would be needed. Anxiety or angina would not preclude a stress test in this case; pulmonary embolus or aortic stenosis are not likely by history and physical.

160. The answer is a. *(Fauci, 14/e, pp 1318–1319.)* The classic symptoms of aortic stenosis are exertional dyspnea, angina pectoris, and syncope. Physical findings include a narrow pulse pressure and the systolic murmur as described in answer A (rather than the aortic insufficiency murmur of answer B, the mitral regurgitation murmur of answer C, or the mitral valve prolapse click of answer D).

161. The answer is a. *(Fauci, 14/e, p 1311.)* The history and physical exam findings are consistent with mitral stenosis. A diastolic rumbling, apical murmur is characteristic. An accentuated first heart sound and opening snap may also be present. The etiology of mitral stenosis is usually rheumatic. It is rarely congenital. Two-thirds of patients afflicted are women.

162. The answer is c. *(Fauci, 14/e, pp 200–201, 1303–1305.)* A holosystolic murmur at the mid-left sternal border is the murmur most characteristic of a ventricular septal defect. Both the murmur of ventricular septal defect and the murmur of mitral regurgitation are enhanced by exercise and diminished by amyl nitrate. Answers A, B, D, and E describe the usual findings in aortic stenosis, atrial septal defect, aortic insufficiency, and patent ductus arteriosus, respectively.

163. The answer is e. *(Fauci, 14/e, p 1262.)* PVCs are common in patients with and without heart disease, detected in 60% of adult males on Holter monitoring. Occasional unifocal PVCs do not suggest any of the underlying diseases described.

164. The answer is e. *(Fauci, 14/e, p 1263.)* Minimally symptomatic PVCs do not require treatment. Antiarrhythmic therapy in this setting has not been shown to reduce sudden cardiac death or overall mortality. A beta blocker would be the best choice if symptoms began to interfere with daily activities.

165. The answer is d. *(Fauci, 14/e, pp 1264–1265.)* In general, in patients with atrial fibrillation, therapeutic anticoagulation with warfarin (Coumadin) reduces the incidence of future stroke to a greater extent than the use of aspirin. This particular patient may be a candidate for medical or electrical cardioversion, which requires pretreatment with Coumadin for two to three weeks (if the atrial fibrillation has been present for over 48 to 72 hours or is of unknown time onset).

166. The answer is c. *(Alexander, 9/e, pp 885–886.)* Paroxysmal supraventricular tachycardia typically displays a narrow QRS complex without clearly discernable P waves, with rate in the 160 to 190 range. The rate is faster in atrial flutter. Atrial fibrillation would show an irregularly irregular rate. Wide QRS complexes would be expected in ventricular tachycardia.

167. The answer is a. *(Aehlert, 1/e, p 258.)* Adenosine is the drug of choice for supraventricular tachycardia, with verapamil the next alternative. Adenosine has an excellent safety profile, making it the preferred drug for supraventricular tachycardia.

168. The answer is g. *(Fauci, 14/e, p 1257.)* This ECG shows Mobitz type I second-degree AV block, also known as *Wenckebach phenomenon,* characterized by progressive PR interval prolongation prior to block of an atrial impulse. This rhythm generally does not require therapy. It may be seen in normal individuals; other causes include inferior MI and drug intoxications such as digoxin, beta blockers, or calcium channel blockers. Even in the post-MI setting, it is usually stable, although it has the potential to progress to higher-degree AV block with consequent need for pacemaker.

169. The answer is d. *(Aehlert, 1/e, pp 20–21.)* One cannot automatically assume initially that the individual had a cardiac or respiratory arrest. Therefore, first determine responsiveness by tapping or gently shaking the victim and shouting, "Are you OK?" Then activate the EMS system. This can then be followed by the ABCs (establishing *airway,* assessing *breathing,* assessing *circulation*).

170. The answer is d. *(Aehlert, 1/e, pp 46 and 253.)* A precordial thump may be administered in a witnessed arrest if a defibrillator is not immediately available. However, the standard approach to ventricular fibrillation or pulseless ventricular tachycardia involves defibrillation with 200 joules, then 300, then 360, followed, if needed, by epinephrine and lidocaine.

171. The answer is b. *(Fauci, 14/e, p 1393.)* Immediate therapy with nitroprusside is indicated, although it would be avoided in the presence of renal insufficiency. Other options include IV nitroglycerin or IV enalaprilat. IV labetalol is often used in hypertensive urgencies, but as a beta blocker is relatively contraindicated in asthma. An oral medication would be difficult in a lethargic patient and slow-acting. Sublingual nifedipine is no longer used due to potential side effects.

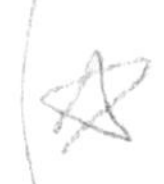

172–173. The answers are 172-b, 173-b. *(Fauci, 14/e, pp 1310–1311.)* This 18-year-old presents with classic features of rheumatic fever. His clinical manifestations include arthritis, fever, murmur. A subcutaneous nodule is noted and a rash of erythema marginatum is described. These subcutaneous nodules are pea-size and usually seen over extensor tendons. The rash is usually pink with clear centers and serpiginous margins. Laboratory data show an elevated erythrocyte sedimentation rate as usually occurs in rheumatic fever. The ECG shows evidence of first-degree AV block. An antistreptolysin O antibody is necessary to diagnose the disease by documenting prior streptococcal infection. Most experts recommend the use of glucocorticoids when carditis is part of the picture of rheumatic fever. Hence, in this patient with first-degree AV block, corticosteroids would be indicated. Penicillin should also be given to eradicate group A beta-hemolytic streptococci.

174. The answer is b. *(Fauci, 14/e, p 1363.)* The ECG in the figure shows complete heart block. P waves and QRS complexes are completely dissociated. Complete heart block in the setting of acute myocardial infarction requires transvenous pacemaker placement.

175. The answer is d. *(Fauci, 14/e, pp 1355–1359.)* The ECG shows acute ST-segment elevations in the anterior precordial leads. The symptoms have persisted for only one hour and the patient does not seem to have any contraindications to thrombolytic therapy, which may be given along with aspirin. Nitroglycerin and morphine are indicated for pain control. Beta blockers reduce pain, limit infarct size, and decrease ventricular arrhythmias. There is no role for digoxin in this acute setting.

176. The answer is c. *(Fauci, 14/e, pp 1242–1244.)* The ECG shows ST-segment elevation in inferior leads II, III, and aVF with reciprocal ST-depression in aVL, consistent with an acute inferior MI. An anterior MI would give ST-segment elevation in the precordial leads. Pericarditis classically gives pleuritic chest pain and diffuse ST-segment elevation (except aVR) on ECG. Costochondritis, esophageal reflux, cholecystitis, and duodenal ulcer disease can all cause the symptoms of substernal chest pain, but not these ECG findings.

177. The answer is a. *(Fauci, 14/e, p 1392.)* The most common cause of refractory hypertension is noncompliance. A history from the patient is useful, and pill count is the best compliance check. Cushing's disease, coarctation, and renal artery stenosis are secondary causes that could result in refractory hypertension, but no clues to these diagnoses are apparent on physical exam.

178. The answer is c. *(Fauci, 14/e, p 1234.)* An S_3 gallop is among the more specific signs of systolic dysfunction, particularly in an older patient. Ankle edema is commonly found in elderly patients secondary to venous insufficiency and other local factors. Wheezes may be present in patients with left ventricular failure, but also occur in asthma and obstructive lung disease.

179. The answer is c. *(Fauci, 14/e, pp 1334–1335.)* The patient's chest pain is most likely due to pericarditis. An enlarged cardiac silhouette without other chest x-ray findings of heart failure suggests pericardial effusion. Echocardiography is the most sensitive, specific way of determining whether pericardial fluid is present. The effusion appears as an echo-free space between the moving epicardium and stationary pericardium. It is unnecessary to perform cardiac catheterization for the purpose of evaluating pericardial effusion. Radionuclide scanning is not a preferred method for demonstrating pericardial fluid.

180. The answer is c. *(Fauci, 14/e, pp 1336–1337.)* The patient has developed cardiac tamponade, a condition in which pericardial fluid under increased pressure impedes diastolic filling, resulting in reduced cardiac output and hypotension. On exam there is elevation of jugular venous pressure. The jugular venous pulse shows a sharp *x* descent, the inward impulse seen at the time of the carotid pulsation. In contrast to pulmonary edema, the lungs are usually clear. Neither a strong apical beat nor an S_3 gallop would be expected in tamponade.

181. The answer is e. *(Alexander, 9/e, pp 1711–1712.)* Cor pulmonale is characterized by the presence of pulmonary hypertension and consequent right ventricular dysfunction. Its causes include diseases leading to hypoxic vasoconstriction, as in cystic fibrosis; occlusion of the pulmonary vasculature, as in pulmonary thromboembolism; and parenchymal destruction, as in sarcoidosis. The right ventricle, in the presence of a chronic increase in afterload, becomes hypertrophic, dilates, and fails. The electrocardiographic findings, as illustrated in the question, include tall, peaked P waves in leads II, III, and aVF, which indicate right atrial enlargement; tall R waves in leads V_1 to V_3 and a deep S wave in V_6 with associated ST-T wave changes, which indicate right ventricular hypertrophy; and right axis deviation. Right bundle branch block occurs in 15% of patients.

182. The answer is c. *(Alexander, 9/e, p 1341.)* Myxomas are histologically benign and account for up to one-half of all cases of primary cardiac tumors. Because they are most commonly located in the left atrium and are pedunculated, they are particularly prone to mimicking mitral stenosis as a result of a ball-valve effect and causing mitral regurgitation due to trauma to the mitral leaflets. Noncardiac manifestations of myxomas include fever, weight loss, arthralgia, and anemia. Surgical excision is curative. Cardiac sarcomas are the most common malignant primary cardiac tumor and are uniformly rapidly fatal.

183. The answer is c. *(Fauci, 14/e, p 1265.)* The rhythm strip exhibited in the question reveals atrial flutter with 4:1 atrioventricular (AV) block. Atrial flutter is characterized by an atrial rate of 280 to 320 per minute; the electrocardiogram typically reveals a sawtooth baseline configuration due to the flutter waves. In the strip presented, every fourth atrial depolarization is conducted through the AV node, resulting in a ventricular rate of 75 per minute.

184. The answer is a. *(Fauci, 14/e, p 1317.)* The fundamental defect in mitral valve prolapse is an abnormality of the valve's connective tissue with secondary proliferation of myxomatous tissue. The redundant leaflet or leaflets prolapse toward the left atrium in systole, which results in the auscultated click and murmur and characteristic echocardiographic findings. Any maneuver that reduces left ventricular size, such as standing or Valsalva, allows the click and murmur to occur earlier in systole; conversely, those maneuvers that increase left ventricular size, such as squatting and propranolol administration, delay the onset of the click and murmur. While most patients with mitral valve prolapse have a benign prognosis, a small percentage die suddenly. Severe mitral regurgitation is an uncommon complication. Antibiotic prophylaxis to prevent endocarditis is recommended for those with typical auscultatory findings, including a systolic murmur. Beta-blocker therapy is reserved for symptoms, including those related to arrhythmias.

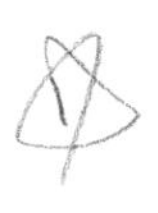

185. The answer is c. *(Alexander, 9/e, p 2207.)* The list of conditions at relatively high risk of development of infective endocarditis includes Marfan's syndrome, prosthetic heart valves, coarctation of the aorta, aortic valve disease, ventricular septal defect, mitral insufficiency, and patent ductus arteriosus. Mitral valve prolapse, pure mitral stenosis, and tricuspid and pulmonary valve disease are among the conditions at intermediate risk. Among the conditions considered to be at very low risk are atrial septal defect, syphilitic aortitis, and cardiac pacemakers.

186. The answer is b. *(Fauci, 14/e, p 1234.)* Normally, the second heart sound (S_2) is composed of aortic closure followed by pulmonic closure. Because inspiration increases blood return to the right side of the heart, pulmonic closure is delayed, which results in normal splitting of S_2 during inspiration. Paradoxical splitting of S_2, however, refers to a splitting of S_2 that is narrowed instead of widened with inspiration consequent to a delayed aortic closure. Paradoxical splitting can result from any electrical or mechanical event that delays left ventricular systole. Thus, aortic stenosis and hypertension, which increase resistance to systolic ejection of blood, delay closure of the aortic valve. Acute ischemia from angina or acute myocardial infarction also can delay ejection of blood from the left ventricle. The most common cause of paradoxical splitting—left bundle branch block—delays electrical activation of the left ventricle. Right bundle branch block results in a wide splitting of S_2 that widens further during inspiration. An S_3 is typically heard with congestive heart failure, an S_4 with

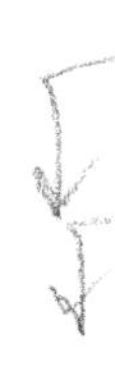

hypertension, an opening snap with mitral stenosis, and a mid-systolic click with mitral valve prolapse.

187–189. The answers are 187-d, 188-b, 189-f. *(Fauci, 14/e, pp 1320–1323 and 1331.)* The diastolic murmur described is characteristic of aortic regurgitation. Unless it is very minor in magnitude, the aortic regurgitant murmur will be accompanied by peripheral signs such as widened pulse pressure. A holosystolic murmur that is increased on inspiration is the result of tricuspid insufficiency. The neck veins are usually distended with prominent *v* waves and signs of right-sided heart failure. The final murmur describes hypertrophic cardiomyopathy, which may also be heard at the apex, where it is more holosystolic.

190–194. The answers are 190-d, 191-c, 192-h, 193-i, 194-b. *(Fauci, 14/e, pp 1363, 1374, 1294, 1363, 1331.)* Sinus bradycardia is a common rhythm disturbance in acute inferior MI, secondary to vagal tone. With associated hypotension, atropine should be given. Intravenous inotropic agents are generally not required.

The syndrome of sudden onset of chest pain at night in association with ST-segment elevation was initially described by Prinzmetal. Classically, the syndrome is caused by coronary artery spasm. Calcium channel blockers are the agents of choice.

ACE inhibitors are active on the arterial bed to reduce impedance to the ejection of blood flow from the left ventricle as well as acting on the venous bed to decrease preload. ACE inhibitors are usually effective in mild as well as severe CHF. A 22% reduction in mortality from progressive heart failure has been found in class II and III heart failure patients. Accelerated idioventricular rhythm develops in up to 25% of post-MI patients. Enhanced automaticity of Purkinje fibers is considered the most likely etiology. At rates less than 90 this is usually considered a benign rhythm and only observation is necessary.

The physical findings described in the final clinical scenario strongly suggest the diagnosis of hypertrophic cardiomyopathy. Digoxin should be avoided in this process. Beta adrenergic agents have been used extensively and are considered the agents of choice, especially in the setting of palpitations. A beneficial effect of calcium channel blockers has sometimes been shown; however, worsening of heart failure can occur.

195–198. The answers are 195-a, 196-b, 197-d, 198-c. *(Fauci, 14/e, p 1234.)* In the normal patient, the second heart sound splits into two components during inspiration and is single during expiration. During inspiration, there is increased venous return to the right ventricle. Severe aortic stenosis may produce expiratory, or paradoxical, splitting. The aortic component is so delayed that it comes after the pulmonic component closure. In inspiration, the delay of P_2 puts the two closure sounds close together.

In right bundle branch block the pulmonary closure sound is delayed, making P_2 more widely split after A_2 than is usual. In an aortic septal defect, the degree of splitting of P_2 is the same during both inspiration and expiration.

199–204. The answers are 199-d, 200-c, 201-a, 202-b, 203-e, 204-g. *(Fauci, 14/e, pp 1387–1388.)* Captopril, by inhibiting the angiotensin converting enzyme, is a potent antihypertensive agent because it prevents the generation of angiotensin II, a vasoconstrictor, and inhibits the degradation of bradykinin, a vasodilator. While especially useful in renovascular hypertension, it may cause membranous glomerulopathy, the nephrotic syndrome, and leukopenia. The most common side effect is cough.

Hydralazine is an arterial vasodilator generally used in conjunction with drugs that prevent reflex sympathetic stimulation of the heart, such as beta blockers and methyldopa. A lupus-like syndrome has been associated with the use of hydralazine.

Propranolol is a nonselective beta blocker and may therefore cause bronchospasm in susceptible patients. Beta blockers, as a class, may reduce HDL cholesterol and increase serum triglyceride levels.

Minoxidil is a more potent vasodilator than hydralazine, but its use is limited by a high incidence of hirsutism. Marked fluid retention may also occur.

Spironolactone, a potassium-sparing diuretic, and methyldopa, a centrally acting antiadrenergic agent, are two antihypertensives that may cause gynecomastia.

Alpha blockers such as terazosin may rarely (in <1%) cause first-dose syncope; they may improve, not cause, urinary retention. Rebound hypertension is associated with clonidine and cyanide toxicity with nitroprusside.

205–208. The answers are 205-e, 206-d, 207-b, 208-a. *(Fauci, 14/e, p 1245.)* Hypokalemia typically increases automaticity of myocardial fibers, which results in ectopic beats or arrhythmias. Electrocardiography in hypokalemia reveals flattening of the T wave and prominent U waves.

Hyperkalemia decreases the rate of spontaneous diastolic depolarization in all pacemaker cells. It also results in slowing of conduction. One of the earliest electrocardiographic signs of hyperkalemia is the appearance of tall, peaked T waves. More severe elevations of the serum potassium result in widening of the QRS complex.

Hypocalcemia results in prolongation of the QT interval. Low serum calcium levels may also be associated with a decrease in myocardial contractility.

At serum sodium levels compatible with life, neither hyponatremia nor hypernatremia results in any characteristic electrocardiographic abnormalities.

ENDOCRINOLOGY AND METABOLIC DISEASE

DIRECTIONS: Each item below contains a question or incomplete statement followed by suggested responses. Select the **one best** response to each question.

Items 209–210

209. A 50-year-old obese female is taking oral hypoglycemic agents. While being treated for an upper respiratory infection, she develops lethargy and is brought to the emergency room. On physical exam, there is no focal neurologic finding or neck rigidity. Laboratory results are as follows:

Na^+	134 meq/L
K^+	4.0 meq/L
HCo_3	25 meq/L
glucose	900 mg/dL
BUN	84 mg/dL
Creatinine	3.0 mg/dL
BP	120/80 sitting
BP	105/65 lying

The most likely cause of this patients coma is

a. Diabetic ketoacidosis
b. Hyperosmolar coma
c. Inappropriate ADH
d. Bacterial meningitis

210. The most important treatment in this patient is

a. Large volumes of fluid, insulin; seek concurrent illnesses
b. Bicarbonate infusion 100 meq/L
c. Rapid glucose lowering with intravenous insulin
d. 30 meq/hr of KCL

211. A 50-year-old female is 5 feet 7 inches and weighs 165 pounds. There is a family history of diabetes mellitus. Fasting blood glucose is 150 mg/dL on two occasions. She is asymptomatic, and physical exam shows no abnormalities. The treatment of choice is

a. Observe
b. Diet and weight reduction
c. Insulin
d. Oral hypoglycemic agent

Items 212–214

212. This 30-year-old female complains of palpitations, fatigue, and insomnia. On physical exam, her extremities are warm and she is tachycardic. There is diffuse thyroid gland enlargement and proptosis. There is an orange thickening of the skin in the pretibial area. Which of the following lab values would you expect in this patient?

a. Increased TSH, total thyroxine, total T_3
b. Decreased TSH, increased total thyroxine
c. Increased T_3 uptake decreased T_3
d. Normal T_4, decreased TSH

213. The cause of this patient's thyrotoxicosis is

a. Autoimmune disease
b. Benign tumor
c. Malignancy
d. Viral infection of the thyroid

214. The treatment of choice in this patient, for whom remission from Graves' disease is possible, is

a. Methimazole
b. Radioactive iodine
c. Thyroid surgery
d. Oral corticosteroids

Items 215–216

215. A 30-year-old female complains of fatigue, constipation, and weight gain. There is no prior history of neck surgery or radiation. Her voice is hoarse and her skin is dry. Serum TSH is elevated and T_4 is low. The most likely cause of these findings is

a. Autoimmune disease
b. Postablative hypothyroidism
c. Pituitary hypofunction
d. Thyroid carcinoma

216. Autoimmune thyroiditis can be confirmed in this patient by

a. Serum for antithyroid peroxidase
b. Antinuclear antibody
c. Thyroid uptake resin
d. Thyroid aspiration

217. On routine physical exam, a young woman is found to have a thyroid nodule. There is no pain, hoarseness, hemoptysis, or local symptoms. Serum TSH is normal. The next step in evaluation would be

a. Ultrasonography
b. Thyroid scan
c. Surgical resection
d. Fine-needle aspiration of thyroid

DIRECTIONS: Each group of questions below consists of lettered headings followed by a set of numbered items. For each numbered item select the **one** lettered heading with which it is most closely associated. Each lettered heading may be used once, more than once, or not at all.

Items 218–220

Match the clinical description with the most likely diagnosis.

a. Acromegaly
b. Prolactin secreting adenoma
c. Cushing's disease
d. Empty sella syndrome
e. TSH-secreting adenoma
f. Diabetes instipidius

218. 30-year-old woman has cervical fat pad, purple striae, hirsutism

219. Irregular menses, galactorrhea in nonpregnant woman, has bitemporal hemianopsia

220. Obese hypertensive woman has chronic headaches, normal pituitary function

DIRECTIONS: Each item below contains a question or incomplete statement followed by suggested responses. Select the **one best** response to each question.

221. What is the best advice to give a middle-aged diabetic male about exercise?

a. Exercise should be avoided because it may cause foot trauma
b. Active lifestyle helps prevent the long-term complications of diabetes
c. Vigorous exercise cannot precipitate hypoglycemia
d. A stress test is a necessity for all diabetics prior to beginning an exercise program

222. A diabetic patient asks for clarification about dietary management. Which of the following is good advice?

a. Restrict carbohydrates and eat a high-protein diet
b. Avoid artificial sweetners
c. Less than 10% of caloric intake should be saturated fat
d. Caloric intake should be very consistent from one day to another

223. A 55-year-old male, as part of a review of systems, describes an inability to achieve erection. The patient has mild diabetes and is on a beta blocker for hypertension. The *first* step in evaluation is

a. Serum testosterone
b. Serum gonadotropin
c. Information about libido and morning erections
d. Papaverine injection

Items 224–226

224. A 90-year-old male complains of hip and back pain. He has also developed headaches, hearing loss, and tinnitus. On physical exam the skull appears enlarged, with prominent superficial veins. There is marked kyphosis and the bones of the leg appear deformed. Plasma alkaline phosphatase is elevated. A skull x-ray shows sharply demarcated lucencies in the frontal, parietal, and occipited bones. X-rays of the hip show thickening of the pelvic brim. The most likely diagnosis is

a. Multiple myeloma
b. Paget's disease
c. Hypercalcemia
d. Metastatic bone disease

225. The etiology of the process has been shown to be

a. Endocrinopathy
b. Viral infection
c. Malignancy
d. Unknown

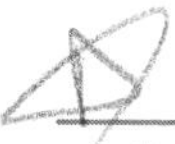

226. The treatment of choice for this patient would be

a. Observation
b. Nonsteroidal anti-inflammatory
c. Calcitonin or bisphosponates
d. Interferon alpha

227. A 50-year-old female is evaluated for hypertension. Her blood pressure is 130/98. She complains of polyuria and of mild muscle weakness. She is on no diuretics or other blood pressure medication. On physical exam the PMI is displaced to the sixth intercostal space. There is no sign of congestive heart failure and no edema.

Laboratory:

Na^+	147 meg/dL
K^+	2.3 meg/dL
Cl^-	112 neg/dL
HCO_3	27 meg/dL

The patient is on no other medication. She does not eat licorice. The first step in diagnosis would be

a. 24-hour urine for cortisol
b. Urinary metanephrine
c. Measure plasma resin and aldosterone
d. Obtain renal angiogram

Items 228–230

228. A 40-year-old alcoholic male is being treated for tuberculosis, but he has not been compliant with his medications. He complains of increasing weakness and fatigue. He appears to have lost weight, and his blood pressure is 80/50 mm Hg. There is increased pigmentation over the elbows. Cardiac exam is normal. The next step in evaluation should be

a. CBC with iron and iron-binding capacity
b. Erythrocyte sedimentation rate
c. Early-morning serum cortisol and cosynotropin stimulation
d. Blood cultures

229. In advanced stage of this disease, the most likely electrolyte abnormalities will be

a. Low serum Na^+
b. Low serum K^+
c. Low serum Na^+ and high serum K^+
d. Low serum K^+

230. The treatment of choice for this patient would be

a. Hydrocortisone once per day
b. Hydrocortisone twice per day plus fludrocortisone
c. Hydrocortisone only during periods of stress
d. Daily ACTH

231. A 60-year-old woman comes to the emergency room in coma. The patient's temperature is 90°F. She is bradycardic. The thyroid gland is enlarged. There is bilateral hyporeflexia. The next step in management would be

a. Await results of T_4, TSH
b. Obtain T_4, TSH; begin thyroid hormone and glucocorticoid
c. Begin rapid rewarming
d. Obtain CT scan of head

232. A 19-year-old with insulin-dependent diabetes mellitus is taking 30 units of NPH insulin each morning and 15 units at night. Because of persistent morning glycosuria with some ketonuria, the evening dose is increased to 20 units. This worsens the morning glycosuria, and now moderate ketones are noted in urine. The patient complains of sweats and headaches at night. The next step in management would be

a. Increase the evening dose of insulin
b. Increase the morning dose of insulin
c. Switch from human NPH to pork insulin
d. Obtain blood sugar levels between 2 and 5 A.M.

233. A 30-year-old woman is found to have a low serum thyroxine level after being evaluated for fatigue. Five years ago she had been treated for Grave's disease with radioactive iodine. The diagnostic test of choice is

a. Serum TSH
b. Serum T_3
c. TRH stimulation test
d. Radioactive iodine uptake

234. A 25-year-old woman is admitted for hypertensive crisis. In the hospital, blood pressure is labile and responds poorly to antihypertensive therapy. The patient complains of palpitations and apprehension. Her past medical history shows that during an operation for appendicitis, she developed hypotension during surgery.

Hct: 49% (37–48)
WBC: 11×10^3mm (4.3–10.8)
Plasma glucose: 160 mg/dL (75–115)
Plasma calcium: 11 mg/dL (9–10.5)

The most likely diagnosis is

a. Pheochromocytoma
b. Renal artery stenosis
c. Essential hypertension
d. Insulin-dependent diabetes mellitus

DIRECTIONS: Each group of questions below consists of lettered headings followed by a set of numbered items. For each numbered item select the **one** lettered heading with which it is most closely associated. Each lettered heading may be used once, more than once, or not at all.

Items 235–237

Match each symptom or sign with the appropriate disease.

a. Subacute thyroiditis
b. Grave's disease
c. Surreptitious hyperthyroidism
d. Multinodular goiter
e. Thyroid nodule

235. Weakness, tremor, heat intolerance. Raised, thickened skin with *peau d'orange* appearance.

236. Weakness, tremor in male nursing assistant. No ophthalmopathy or skin lesions. RAIU shows subnormal values. T_4 elevated.

237. Thyroid tender, erythrocyte sedimentation rate elevated, heat intolerance.

DIRECTIONS: Each item below contains a question or incomplete statement followed by suggested responses. Select the **one best** response to each question.

238. The patient pictured below complains of persistent headache. Her most likely visual field defect would be

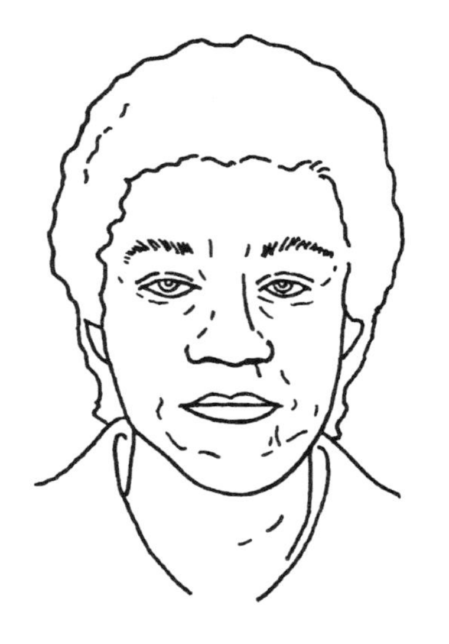

a. Bitemporal hemianopsia
b. Unilateral blindness
c. Left homonymous hemianopsia
d. Right homonymous hemianopsia

239. A patient with small cell carcinoma of the lung develops lethargy. Serum electrolytes are drawn and show a serum sodium of 118 mg/L. There is no evidence of edema, orthostatic hypotension, or dehydration. Urine is concentrated with an osmolality of 320 mmol/kg. Serum BUN, creatinine, and glucose are within normal range. Which of the following is the next appropriate step?

a. Normal saline infusion
b. Diuresis
c. Fluid restriction
d. Tetracycline

240. A 40-year-old woman complains of weakness and amenorrhea. She has hypertension and diabetes mellitus. Picture is shown below. The clinical findings may be explained by

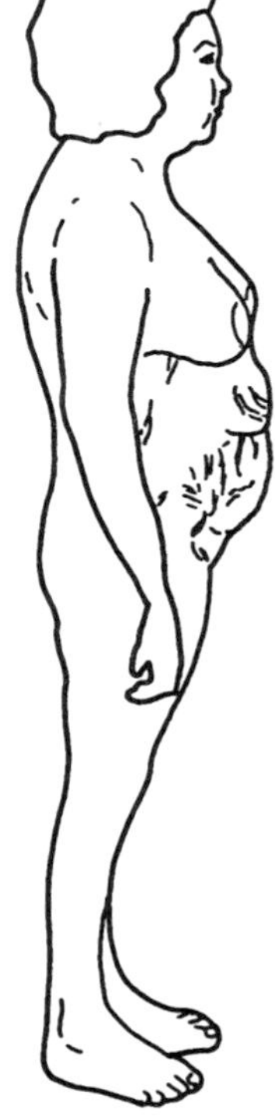
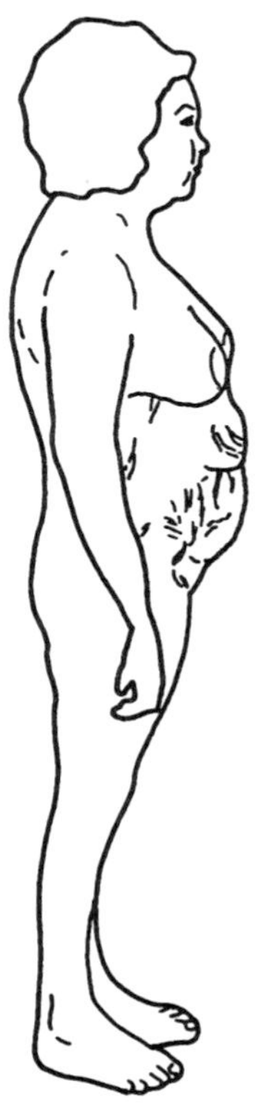

a. Pituitary tumor
b. Adrenal tumor
c. Ectopic ACTH production
d. Any of the above

241. The patient pictured below presents with gynecomastia and infertility. On exam, he has small, firm testes. Which of the following is correct?

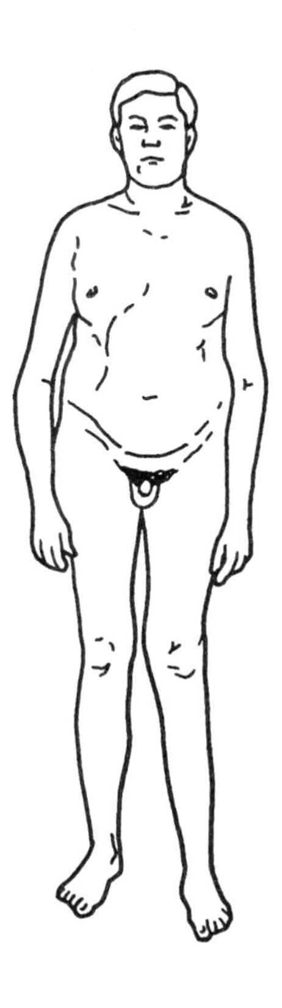

a. The patient is likely to have low levels of gonadotropins
b. The patient has Turner's syndrome
c. His most likely karyotype is 47 XXY
d. The patient will have normal sperm count and testosterone level

242. A 52-year-old man complains of impotence. On physical examination, he has an elevated jugular venous pulse, S_3 gallop, and hepatomegaly. He also appears tanned, with pigmentation along joint folds. His left knee is swollen and tender. The plasma glucose is 250 mg/dL, and liver enzymes are elevated. Your next study to establish the diagnosis should be

a. Detection of nocturnal penile tumescence
b. Determination of serum ferritin
c. Determination of serum copper
d. Detection of hepatitis B surface antigen
e. Echocardiography

243. A 30-year-old man is evaluated for a thyroid nodule. The patient reports that his father died from thyroid cancer and that a brother had a history of recurrent renal stones. Blood calcitonin concentration is 2000 pg/mL (normal: less than 100); serum calcium and phosphate levels are normal. Before referring the patient to a surgeon, the physician should

a. Obtain a liver scan
b. Perform a calcium infusion test
c. Measure urinary catecholamines
d. Administer suppressive doses of thyroxine and measure levels of thyroid-stimulating hormone
e. Treat the patient with radioactive iodine

244. A 32-year-old woman has a three-year history of oligomenorrhea that has progressed to amenorrhea during the past year. She has observed loss of breast fullness, reduced hip measurements, acne, increased body hair, and deepening of her voice. Physical examination reveals frontal balding, clitoral hypertrophy, and a male escutcheon. Urinary free cortisol and dehydroepiandrosterone sulfate (DHEAS) are normal. Her plasma testosterone level is 6 ng/mL (normal: 0.2 to 0.8). The most likely diagnosis of this patient's disorder is

a. Cushing's syndrome
b. Arrhenoblastoma
c. Polycystic ovary syndrome
d. Granulosa-theca cell tumor

245. A 54-year-old man who has had a Billroth II procedure for peptic ulcer disease now presents with abdominal pain and is found to have recurrent ulcer disease. The physician is considering this patient's illness to be secondary either to a retained antrum or to a gastrinoma. Which of the following tests would best differentiate the two conditions?

a. Random gastrin level
b. Determination of 24-h acid production
c. Serum calcium level
d. Secretin infusion
e. Insulin-induced hypoglycemia

246. A 55-year-old woman who has a history of severe depression and who had radical mastectomy for carcinoma of the breast one year previously develops polyuria, nocturia, and excessive thirst. Laboratory values are as follows:

Serum electrolytes (meq/L): [qlNa$^+$ 149; K$^+$ 3.6
Serum calcium: 9.5 mg/dL
Blood glucose: 110 mg/dL
Blood urea nitrogen: 30 mg/dL
Urine osmolality: 150 mOsm/kg

The most likely diagnosis is

a. Psychogenic polydipsia
b. Renal glycosuria
c. Hypercalciuria
d. Diabetes insipidus
e. Inappropriate antidiuretic hormone syndrome

ENDOCRINOLOGY AND METABOLIC DISEASE

Answers

209. The answer is b. *(Stobo, 23/e, pp 328–329.)* This obese patient on oral hypoglycemics has developed hyperglycemia and lethargy during an upper respiratory infection. The patient's serum osmolality is as follows:

$$\frac{900}{18}\text{ (glucose)} + 2\ (\text{Na}^+ + \text{K}^+) + \frac{84}{2.8} = 50 + 276 + 30 = 356$$

Hence the serum osmolality is greater than 350 mOsm/kg. The serum bicarbonate is too high to be consistent with diabetic ketoacidosis. The hyponatremia is related to hyperglycemia. SIADH could not be diagnosed in this clinical setting. The patient's diabetes likely went out of control due to infection. There is no clinical evidence for meningitis.

210. The answer is a. *(Stobo, 23/e, pp 328–329.)* The primary treatment for hyperosmolar nonketotic states is fluid replacement, usually normal saline. Hypotonic saline may be given for severe hypernatremia or congestive heart failure. Hyperglycemia can be corrected slowly. The patient is not acidotic and would not require bicarbonate treatment (used in severe DKA when pH is less than 7.0). The patient's serum potassium is in the normal range and would not be expected to fall rapidly.

211. The answer is b. *(Stobo, 23/e, pp 324–330.)* The primary treatment for type 2 diabetes is dietary. About half of all patients can maintain a normal blood sugar with weight reduction. If weight reduction fails, a number of oral hypoglycemics are available as the next step.

212. The answer is b. *(Stobo, 23/e, pp 293–298.)* This patient has clinical symptoms of thyrotoxicosis. Most patients with thyrotoxicosis have increases in total and free concentrations of T_3 and T_4. (Some may have isolated T_3 or T_4 increases.) Most thyrotoxicosis results in suppression of pituitary TSH secretion, so low TSH levels can also confirm the diagnosis.

213. The answer is a. *(Stobo, 23/e, pp 293–298.)* This patient has, in addition to thyrotoxicosis, orbitopathy as well as the characteristic dermopathy of Graves' disease called *pretibial myxedema*. Graves' disease is an autoimmune phenomena. Biopsy of the thyroid shows lymphocytic infiltration. Toxic multinodular goiter produces thyrotoxicosis caused by benign, functionally autonomous tumors. It would not produce the proptosis or dermopathy of Graves' disease. Subacute thyroiditis (de Quervain's) is probably caused by a viral infection. It produces a transient hyperthyroidism followed by hypothyroidism.

214. The answer is a. *(Stobo, 23/e, pp 297–298.)* Antithyroid drugs are considered by most to be the treatment of choice in a patient with Graves' disease. Surgical thyroidectomy is usually reserved for those with thyroid malignancy or thyrotoxic pregnant women who have had severe side effects to medication. Iodine-131 has been used successfully in Graves' disease, but often causes permanent hypothyroidism.

215. The answer is a. *(Stobo, 23/e, pp 298–302.)* In primary hypothyroidism, autoimmune thyroiditis is the most common insult. Primary hypothyroidism can result from surgery or radiation therapy, but there is no such history in this patient. Thyroid cancer does not cause hypothyroidism.

216. The answer is a. *(Stobo, 23/e, pp 298–299.)* Autoimmune thyroiditis can be confirmed by serum antithyroid peroxidase (which was formerly called antimicrosomal antibody) and by measuring antithyroglobulin antibody.

217. The answer is d. *(Stobo, 23/e, pp 300–301.)* Thyroid fine-needle biopsy now plays a central role in the differential diagnosis of thyroid nodules. Thyroid scan can show a hot nodule, which would be reassuring that the nodule is benign; a biopsy would be necessary for the cold nodules. Thyroid sonography seldom can rule out malignancy in palpable nodules. Surgery would be indicated if the aspiration biopsy shows malignancy or, in most cases, if it is indeterminate.

218–220. The answers are 218-c, 219-b, 220-d. *(Stobo, 23/e, pp 274–292.)* Cushing's disease produces hypercortisolism secondary to excessive excretion of pituitary ACTH. It often affects women in their childbearing years. Cervical fat pad, purple striae, and hirsutism are characteristic features, as well as muscle wasting, easy bruising, amenorrhea, and psychiatric disturbances. Prolactinoma, or prolactin-secreting adenoma, may cause bitemporal hemianopsia—as all pituitary tumors can. Galactorrhea (lactation not associated with pregnancy) and irregular menses or amenorrhea are the clinical clues. Serum prolactin levels are usually over 250 ng/mL, often distinguishing them from other causes of hyperprolactinemia such as renal failure. Empty sella syndrome is enlargement of the sella turcica from CSF pressure compressing the pituitary gland. It is likely to occur in obese, hypertensive women. There are no focal findings. Some women have chronic headaches; others are asymptomatic. MRI will distinguish this syndrome from a pituitary tumor.

221. The answer is b. *(Stobo, 23/e, p 325.)* An active lifestyle and good exercise program can prevent the complications of diabetes. However, there are pitfalls to such a program. Some forms of exercise might jeopardize adequate foot care. Exercise can potentiate hypoglycemia by potentiating insulin action. Diabetics who have other risk factors for cardiovascular disease such as hypertension and hyperlipidemia should have an exercise stress test prior to engaging in a rigorous exercise program.

222. The answer is c. *(Stobo, 23/e, pp 321–331.)* In order to reduce plasma cholesterol and decrease the risk of vascular disease, fat intake should be moderated, with less than 10% of total caloric intake being saturated fat. Caloric distribution does not restrict or decrease carbohydrates. Dietary protein should be moderated, and in patients with diabetic nephropathy, reducing dietary protein is often recommended. Patients with diabetes are usually advised to use artificial sweetners rather than concentrated sweets.

223. The answer is c. *(Stobo, 23/e, pp 309–310.)* The first step in the evaluation of impotence is a complete and detailed history—including libido, ability to attain erection unrelated to sexual intercourse. Loss of all erectile function suggests an organic cause for the disease. In this patient impotence may be the result of depression from the antihypertensive agent or a direct effect of the beta blocker on sexual performance. Diabetes may cause impotence as an effect on penile blood supply or parasympathetic nervous system function. A decrease in libido would suggest testosterone deficiency. Serum testosterone should then be measured and, if low, serum gonadotropins should be measured. In a diabetic with claudication or abnormal femoral pulses, injection of papaverine into the corpora cavernosa can test vascular insufficiency as the cause of impotence. A normal response is an erection within 10 minutes.

224. The answer is b. *(Stobo, 23/e, pp 319–320.)* This patient has widespread Paget's disease of bone. Excessive resorption of bone is followed by replacement of normal marrow with dense, trabecular disorganized bone. Hearing loss and tinnitus is due to direct involvement of the ossicles of the inner ear. Plasma alkaline phosphatase levels represent increased bone turnover. Neither myeloma or metastatic bone disease would result in bony deformity such as skull enlargement.

225. The answer is d. *(Stobo, 23/e, pp 319–320.)* The cause of Paget's disease remains unknown. Some intranuclear inclusions resemble the nucleocapsids of viruses. Measles and respiratory syncytial virus mRNA appears similar to mRNA found in nucleocapsids. No known endocrinopathy has been suggested, and the disease does not involve malignant cells.

226. The answer is c. *(Fauci, 14/e, pp 2266–2268.)* Bone pain, hearing loss, and bony deformity are all indications for specific therapy beyond just the symptomatic relief of nonsteroidal anti-inflammatory agents. Calcitonin restores normal bone modeling. Bisphosphonates bind to hydroxyapatite crystals to decrease bone turnover.

227. The answer is c. *(Stobo, 23/e, pp 288–290.)* The patient has diastolic hypertension with associated hypokalemia. She is not taking diuretics. There is no edema on physical exam. Excessive inappropriate aldosterone production will produce a hypertension with hypokalemia syndrome. Hypersecretion of aldosterone increases distal tubular exchange of sodium for potassium with progressive depletion of body potassium. The hypertension is due to increased sodium absorption. Very low plasma renin that fails to increase with appropriate stimulus (such as volume depletion) and hypersecretion of aldosterone suggest the diagnosis of primary hyperaldosteronism. Suppressed resin activity occurs in about 25% of hypertensive patients with essential hypertension. Lack of suppression of aldosterone is also necessary to diagnose primary aldosteronism. High aldosterone levels that are not suppressed by saline loading prove that there is a primary inappropriate secretion of aldosterone.

228. The answer is c. *(Stobo, 23/e, pp 286–288.)* This patient's symptoms of weakness, fatigue, and weight loss in combination with signs of hypotension and extensor hyperpigmentation are all consistent with Addison's disease. Tuberculosis can involve the adrenal glands and result in adrenal insufficiency. Measurement of serum cortisol baseline and then stimulation with ACTH will confirm the clinical suspicion.

229. The answer is c. *(Stobo, 23/e, pp 286–288.)* Hyponatremia is due to loss of sodium in the urine (aldosterone deficiency) and movement intracellularly. Hyperkalemia is due to aldosterone deficiency, impaired glomerular filtration, and acidosis.

230. The answer is b. *(Stobo, 23/e, pp 286–288.)* Hydrocortisone is the mainstay of treatment. Two-thirds of the dose is taken in the morning and one-third at night in order to approach normal diurnal variation. The mineralocorticoid component of adrenal hormones also needs to be replaced. During periods of intercurrent stress or illness, higher doses of both glucocorticoid and mineralocorticoid are required.

231. The answer is b. *(Stein, 5/e, pp 1810–1811.)* The clinical concern in this patient is myxedema coma. Once this diagnosis is considered, treatment must be started, as it is a medical emergency. Treatment is initiated, and should lab results, when they return, not support the diagnosis, then treatment would be stopped. An intravenous bolus of thyroxine is given (300 to 500 μg), followed by daily intravenous doses. Glucorticoids are given concomitantly. Intravenous fluids are also needed; rewarming should be accompanied slowly, so as not to precipitate cardiac arrhythmias. If alveolar ventilation is compromised, than intubation may also be necessary.

232. The answer is d. *(Stein, 5/e, p 1861.)* Episodic hypoglycemia at night is followed by rebound hyperglycemia. This response, called the *Somogyi phenomena,* develops in response to excessive insulin administration. An adenergic response to hypoglycemia results in increased glycogenolysis, gluconeogenesis, and diminished glucose uptake by peripheral tissues. After documenting hypoglycemia, the insulin dosages are slowly reduced.

233. The answer is a. *(Stein, 5/e, pp 1808–1811.)* TSH levels are always increased in patients with untreated hypothyroidism (from primary thyroid disease) and would be the test of choice in this patient. Serum T_3 is not sensitive for hypothyroidism. The TRH stimulation test is useful in some cases of hyperthyroidism. A decreased RAIU is of limited value because of the low value for lower limit of normal. In goitrous hypothyroidism, the RAIU may even be increased.

234. The answer is a. *(Stein, 5/e, pp 1828–1831.)* A hypertensive crisis in this young woman suggests a secondary cause of hypertension. In the setting of palpitations, apprehension, and hyperglycemia, pheochromocytoma should be considered. Unexplained hypotension associated with surgery or trauma may also suggest the disease. The patient's hypoglycemia is a result of a catecholamine effect of insulin suppression and stimulation of hepatic glucose output. Hypercalcemia has been attributed to ectopic secretion of parathormone-related protein. Renal artery stenosis can cause severe hypertension but would not explain the systemic symptoms or laboratory abnormalities in this case.

235–237. The answers are 235-b, 236-c, 237-a. *(Fauci, 14/e, pp 2012–2033.)* Symptoms of hyperthyroidism with skin involvement characteristic of pretibial myxedema suggest Graves' disease. Skin and eye involvement in association with hyperthyroid symptoms do not occur in hyperthyroidism other than Graves' disease.

Surreptitious hyperthyroidism can occur in health care workers who have access to thyroid hormone. Classic symptoms of hyperthyroidism occur and the serum T_4 is elevated. The radioactive iodine uptake would show subnormal values, as there is no increased thyroid uptake in the gland itself.

A tender thyroid gland and elevated ESR make thyroiditis the likely diagnosis. Hyperthyroid symptoms are common early in the illness.

238. The answer is a. *(Fauci, 14/e, pp 1980–1983.)* The patient shows excessive growth of soft tissue that has resulted in coarsening of facial features, prognathism, and frontal bossing—all characteristic of acromegaly. This growth hormone–secreting pituitary tumor will result in bitemporal hemianopsia when the tumor impinges on the optic chiasm, which lies just above the sella turcica.

239. The answer is c. *(Fauci, 14/e, pp 268–269.)* The patient described has hyponatremia, normovolemia, and a concentrated urine. These features are sufficient to make a diagnosis of inappropriate antidiuretic hormone secretion. Inappropriate ADH secretion occurs by ectopic production from neoplastic tissue. Treatment necessitates restriction of fluid intake. A negative water balance results in rise in serum Na^+ and serum osmolality and symptom improvement.

240. The answer is d. *(Fauci, 14/e, pp 2042–2046.)* The clinical findings all suggest an excess production of cortisol by the adrenal gland. Hypertension, truncal obesity, and abdominal striae are common physical findings. The process responsible for continued excess could be any of those listed—an ACTH-secreting pituitary tumor, an ectopic ACTH-producing neoplasm, and a primary adrenal tumor.

241. The answer is c. *(Fauci, 14/e, pp 2120–2121.)* The picture of infertility, gynecomastia, and tall stature are consistent with Klinefelter's syndrome and an XXY karyotype. The patient has abnormal gonadal development with hyalinized testes that result in low testosterone levels and elevated levels of gonadotropin. Turner's syndrome refers to the 45 karyotype that results in the abnormal sexual organ development in a female.

242. The answer is b. *(Fauci, 14/e, p 2151.)* Iron overload should be considered among patients who present with any one or a combination of the following: hepatomegaly, weakness, pigmentation, atypical arthritis, diabetes, impotence, unexplained chronic abdominal pain, or cardiomyopathy. Excessive alcohol intake increases the diagnostic probability. Diagnostic suspicions should be particularly high when the family history is positive for similar clinical findings. The most frequent cause of iron overload is a common genetic disorder known as (idiopathic) hemochromatosis. Secondary iron storage problems can occur in a variety of anemias. The most practical screening test is the determination of serum iron, transferrin saturation, and plasma ferritin. Plasma ferritin values above 300 ng/mL in males and 200 ng/mL in females suggest increased iron stores, and definitive diagnosis can be done by liver biopsy. Determination of serum copper is needed when Wilson's disease is the probable cause of hepatic abnormalities. The clinical picture here is inconsistent with that diagnosis. Nocturnal penile tumescence and echocardiogram can confirm clinical findings but will not help to establish the diagnosis.

243. The answer is c. *(Fauci, 14/e, pp 2030–2031, 2057, 2228–2229.)* For the patient described in the question, the markedly increased calcitonin levels indicate the diagnosis of medullary carcinoma of the thyroid. In view of the family history, the patient most likely has multiple endocrine neoplasia (MEN) type II, which includes medullary carcinoma of the thyroid gland, pheochromocytoma, and parathyroid hyperplasia. Pheochromocytoma may exist without sustained hypertension, as indicated by excessive urinary catecholamines. Before thyroid surgery is performed on this patient, a pheochromocytoma must be ruled out through urinary catecholamine determinations; the presence of such a tumor might expose him to a hypertensive crisis during surgery. The entire thyroid gland must be removed because foci of parafollicular cell hyperplasia, a premalignant lesion, may be scattered throughout the gland. Successful removal of the medullary carcinoma can be monitored with serum calcitonin levels. Hyperparathyroidism, while unlikely in this patient, is probably present in his brother.

244. The answer is b. *(Fauci, 14/e, p 20.)* The symptoms of masculinization (e.g., alopecia, deepening of voice, clitoral hypertrophy) in the patient presented in the question are characteristic of active androgen-producing tumors. Such extreme virilization is very rarely observed in polycystic ovary syndrome or in Cushing's syndrome; moreover, the presence of normal cortisol and markedly elevated plasma testosterone levels indicates an ovarian rather than adrenal cause of her findings. Arrhenoblastomas are the most common androgen-producing ovarian tumors. Their incidence is highest during the reproductive years. Composed of varying proportions of Leydig's and Sertoli cells, they are generally benign. In contrast to arrhenoblastomas, granulosa-theca cell tumors produce feminization, not virilization.

245. The answer is d. *(Fauci, 14/e, pp 1613–1615, 1582.)* The diagnosis of gastrinoma should be considered in all patients with either recurrent ulcers after surgical correction for peptic ulcer disease, ulcers in the distal duodenum or jejunum, ulcer disease associated with diarrhea, or evidence suggestive of the multiple endocrine neoplasia (MEN) type I (familial association of pituitary, parathyroid, and pancreatic tumors) in ulcer patients. Because basal serum gastrin and basal acid production may both be normal or only slightly elevated in patients with gastrinomas, provocative tests may need to be employed for diagnosis. Both the secretin and calcium infusion tests are used; a paradoxical increase in serum gastrin concentration is seen in response to both infusions in patients with gastrinomas. In contrast, other conditions associated with hypergastrinemia, such as duodenal ulcers, retained antrum, gastric outlet obstruction, antral G-cell hyperplasia, and pernicious anemia, will respond with either no change or a decrease in serum gastrin.

246. The answer is d. *(Fauci, 14/e, p 2004.)* Metastatic tumors rarely cause diabetes insipidus, but of the tumors that may cause it, carcinoma of the breast is by far the most common. In the patient discussed in the question, the diagnosis of diabetes insipidus is suggested by hyponatremia and a low urine osmolality. Psychogenic polydipsia is an unlikely diagnosis since serum sodium is usually mildly reduced in this condition. Renal glycosuria would be expected to induce a higher urine osmolality than this patient has because of the osmotic effect of glucose. While nephrocalcinosis secondary to hypercalcemia may produce polyuria, hypercalciuria does not. Finally, the findings of inappropriate antidiuretic hormone syndrome are the opposite of those observed in diabetes insipidus and thus are incompatible with the clinical picture in this patient.

GASTROENTEROLOGY

DIRECTIONS: Each item below contains a question or incomplete statement followed by suggested responses. Select the **one best** response to each question.

247. A 35-year-old alcoholic male is admitted for nausea, vomiting, and abdominal pain that radiates to the back. A laboratory value that suggests poor prognosis in this patient is

a. Elevated serum lipase
b. Low serum amylase
c. Leukocytosis of 20,000/mm^3
d. Blood pressure, diastolic greater than 90 mm Hg

DIRECTIONS: Each group of questions below consists of lettered headings followed by a set of numbered items. For each numbered item select the **one** lettered heading with which it is most closely associated. Each lettered heading may be used once, more than once, or not at all.

Items 248–250

Match the patient described with the most likely diagnosis.

a. Acute diverticulitis
b. Acute pancreatitis
c. Acute cholecystitis
d. Intestinal bowel syndrome
e. Irritable bowel syndrome
f. Carcinoma of the stomach
g. Acute mesenteric ischemia

248. Colicky RUQ abdominal pain; pain at the inferior angle of the scapula

249. Left lower quadrant pain with history of constipation, leukocytosis

250. Periumbilical pain, distention, vomiting, obstipation

DIRECTIONS: Each item below contains a question or incomplete statement followed by suggested responses. Select the **one best** response to each question.

Items 251–253

251. A 40-year-old cigarette smoker complains of epigastric pain, localized, nonradiating, and described as burning. The pain is partially relieved by eating. There is no weight loss. There has been no use of nonsteroidal anti-inflammatory agents. The pain has been worsening over several months. The most sensitive way to make a specific diagnosis is

a. Barium x-ray
b. Endoscopy
c. Serologic test for *Helicobacter pylori*
d. Serum gastrin

252. This patient is found to have a duodenal ulcer by duodenoscopy. The likelihood of this patient having *H. pylori* in the gastric antrum is

a. 10 to 25%
b. 50%
c. 100%
d. Not known

253. The best way to eradicate *H. pylori* in this patient would be

a. Histamine H_2 receptor antagonist
b. Proton pump inhibitor
c. Amoxicillin, metronidazole, bismuth
d. Misoprostol

Items 254–255

254. A 70-year-old male presents with a complaint of fatigue. There is no history of alcohol abuse or liver disease; the patient is on no medication. Scleral icterus is noted on physical exam. There is no evidence for chronic liver disease on physical exam, and the liver and spleen are nonpalpable. The patient is noted to have a normocytic, nomochromic anemia. The first step in evaluation of this patient would be

a. CT scan of the abdomen
b. Hepatitis profile
c. Liver function tests, including direct versus indirect bilirubin and urine bilirubin
d. Abdominal ultrasound

255. The patient above is noted to have conjugated hyperbilirubinema, with bilirubin detected in the urine. Serum bilirubin 12 mg/dL, AST and ALT in normal range, and alkaline phosphatase 300 U/L. The next step in evaluation would be

a. Ultrasound or CT scan
b. Hepatitis profile
c. Reticulocyte count
d. Family history for hemochromatosis

Items 256–258

256. A 40-year-old male with long-standing alcohol abuse complains of abdominal swelling, which has been progressive over several months. He has a history of gastrointestinal bleeding. On physical exam there are spider angiomata and palmer erythema. Abdominal collateral vessels are seen around the umbilicus. There is shifting dullness, and bulging flanks are noted. An important first step in the patient's evaluation would be

a. Paracentesis, diagnostic
b. UGI series
c. Ethanol level
d. CT scan

257. A paracentesis is performed on the patient previously described. The serum albumin minus ascitic fluid albumin equals 1.2 g/dL. The most likely diagnosis is

a. Portal hypertension
b. Pancreatitis
c. Tuberculous peritonitis
d. Hematoma

258. While hospitalized, the patient's mental status deteriorates. He has been having guaiac-positive stools and a low-grade fever. He also has received sedation for agitation. On physical exam the patient is confused. He has no meningeal signs and no focal neurologic findings. There is hyperreflexia and a nonrhythmic flapping tremor of the wrist. The *most likely* explanation for the mental status change is

a. Tuberculosis meningitis
b. Subdural hematoma
c. Alcohol withdrawal seizure
d. Hepatic encephalopathy

259. A 50-year-old black male with a history of alcohol and tobacco abuse has complained of difficulty swallowing solid food for the past two months. More recently, swallowing fluids has also become a problem. He has noted black, tarry stools on occasion. The patient has lost 10 pounds. Which of the following statements is correct?

a. The patient's prognosis is good
b. Barium contrast study is indicated
c. The most likely tumor is an adenocarcinoma
d. The patient has achalasia

260. A 20-year-old female develops bloody diarrhea while traveling in Mexico. A stool smear shows many polymorphonuclear leukocytes. The most likely diagnosis in this patient is

a. Shigella
b. Rotavirus
c. Norwalk agent
d. *Entamoeba histolytica*

261. A 50-year-old male presents with jaundice, right upper quadrant tenderness, spider angiomata, and ascites. He takes no medication but has been drinking alcohol heavily. Which of the following would be most likely in this patient?

a. Jugular venous distention on physical examination
b. SGPT (ALT) much higher than the SGOT (AST)
c. Mallory bodies on liver biopsy
d. Rapid clinical recovery after abstinence

262. A nursing student has just completed her hepatitis B vaccine series. On reviewing her laboratory studies and assuming she has no prior exposure to hepatitis B, you would expect

a. Positive test for hepatitis B surface antigen
b. Antibody against hepatitis B surface antigen (anti-HB5) alone
c. Antibody against hepatitis core antigen (anti-HBC)
d. Antibody against both surface and core antigen
e. Antibody against hepatitis E antigen

DIRECTIONS: Each group of questions below consists of lettered headings followed by a set of numbered items. For each numbered item select the **one** lettered heading with which it is most closely associated. Each lettered heading may be used once, more than once, or not at all.

Items 263–265

Match the clinical description with the most likely disease process.

a. Primary biliary cirrhosis
b. Sclerosing cholangitis
c. Anaerobic liver abscess
d. Hepatoma
e. Hepatitis C
f. Hepatitis D
g. Hemochromatosis

263. A 40-year-old white female complains of pruritus. Has elevated alkaline phosphatase and positive antimitochondrial antibody.

264. A 70-year-old male with long history of diverticulitis has low-grade fever, elevated alkaline phosphatase, and right upper quadrant pain.

265. A 30-year-old male with ulcerative colitis develops jaundice, pruritus, and right upper quadrant pain. Liver biopsy shows an inflammatory obliterative process affecting intrahepatic and extrahepatic bile ducts.

DIRECTIONS: Each item below contains a question or incomplete statement followed by suggested responses. Select the **one best** response to each question.

266. A 40-year-old male has a history of three duodenal ulcers with prompt recurrence. Symptoms have been associated with severe diarrhea. One of the ulcers occurred close to the jejunum. Serum gastrin levels have been 200 pg/ml. The most useful test in this patient is

a. Colonoscopy
b. Endoscopic retrograde cholangiogram
c. CT scan of abdomen
d. Secretin injection test
e. Upper gastrointestinal series

267. A 40-year-old white male complains of weakness, weight loss, and abdominal pain. On examination the patient has diffuse hyperpigmentation and a palpable liver edge. A polyarthritis of wrist and hips is also noted. Fasting blood sugar is 185 mg/dl. The most likely diagnosis is

a. Insulin-dependent diabetes mellitus
b. Pancreatic carcinoma
c. Addison's disease
d. Hemochromatosis

DIRECTIONS: Each group of questions below consists of lettered headings followed by a set of numbered items. For each numbered item select the **one** lettered heading with which it is most closely associated. Each lettered heading may be used once, more than once, or not at all.

Items 268–270

Match the clinical description with the most likely disease process.

a. Hemolysis secondary to G6PD deficiency
b. Pancreatic carcinoma
c. Acute viral hepatitis
d. Crigler-Najjar syndrome
e. Gilbert's syndrome
f. Cirrhosis of liver

268. Black male develops mild jaundice while being treated for a urinary tract infection. No urine bilirubin. Serum bilirubin is 3 mg/dL—unconjugated. Hemoglobin is 7.

269. A 60-year-old male is noted to have mild jaundice and weight loss. Alkaline phosphatase is very elevated. He's had very pale stools.

270. A young woman complains of fatigue, change in skin color, dark brown urine. She has right upper quadrant tenderness and ALT of 400 (normal: 8 to 20).

DIRECTIONS: Each item below contains a question or incomplete statement followed by suggested responses. Select the **one best** response to each question.

271. Which of the following serological patterns is most consistent with chronic active hepatitis due to hepatitis B?

a. Hepatitis B surface antigen (HBsAg) positive, hepatitis B surface antibody (HBsAb) negative
b. HBsAg negative, hepatitis B core antibody (HBcAb) positive, HBsAb negative
c. Hepatitis B e antigen (HBeAg) negative
d. HBsAg negative, HBcAb negative, hepatitis BsAb positive
e. Hepatitis BsAg negative, HBcAb positive, hepatitis BsAb positive

272. Chronic pancreatitis frequently produces

a. Diabetes mellitus
b. Malabsorption of fat-soluble vitamins D and K
c. Guaiac-positive stool
d. Courvoisier's sign

273. *Clostridium difficile* infection is reliably diagnosed by

a. Identification of *Clostridium difficile* toxin in the stool
b. Isolation of *Clostridium difficile* in a stool culture
c. Stool positive for white blood cells
d. Detection of IgG antibodies against *Clostridium difficile* in the serum

DIRECTIONS: Each group of questions below consists of lettered headings followed by a set of numbered items. For each numbered item select the **one** lettered heading with which it is most closely associated. Each lettered heading may be used once, more than once, or not at all.

Items 274–277

For each histological abnormality found on liver biopsy, select the liver disease with which it is associated

a. Schistosomiasis
b. Primary biliary cirrhosis
c. Alpha$_1$ antitrypsin deficiency
d. Hemochromatosis
e. Alcoholic hepatitis

274. Steatosis

275. Pipestem fibrosis

276. Paucity of bile ducts

277. PAS (periodic acid–Schiff)-positive granules

Items 278–281

For each laboratory test or set of tests, choose the hepatobiliary disease in which it is most likely to be abnormal.

a. Sclerosing cholangitis
b. Primary biliary cirrhosis
c. Autoimmune hepatitis, type 1
d. Wilson's disease
e. Hemochromatosis

278. Antinuclear antibodies (ANA)

279. Ceruloplasmin

280. Serum iron, total iron-binding capacity (TIBC), ferritin

281. Antimitochondrial antibodies

Items 282–285

For each of the following physical findings, select the liver disease with which it is most closely associated.

a. Wilson's disease
b. Alpha$_1$ antitrypsin disease
c. Primary biliary cirrhosis
d. Dubin-Johnson syndrome
e. Hemochromatosis

282. Xanthomas

283. Sunflower cataracts

284. Bronzing of the skin

285. Kayser-Fleischer rings

GASTROENTEROLOGY

Answers

247. The answer is c. *(Fauci, 14/e, pp 1743–1744.)* The Ranson criteria are used to determine prognosis in acute pancreatitis. Factors that adversely affect survival include age greater than 55 years, leukocytosis greater than 16,000 mm^3, glucose greater than 200 mg/dL, LDH greater than 400 IU, AST greater than 250 IU/L. During the initial 48 hours, a fall in hematocrit, hypercalcemia, hypoxemia, increase in BUN, and hypoalbuminemia are also poor prognostic findings. Hypotension with systolic BP less than 90 mm Hg is also a poor prognostic sign; diastolic hypertension is not correlated with prognosis.

248–250. The answers are 248-c, 249-a, 250-d. *(Stobo, 23/e, pp 439–451.)* Right upper quadrant colicky pain is the typical presentation for acute cholecytitis. As a stone passes through the cystic duct, pain may be felt at the right scapula and shoulder. Diverticulitis most commonly presents as pain in the left lower quadrant. It is usually associated with fever and leukocytosis distinguishing it from irritable bowel syndrome. Intestinal obstruction is characterized by periumbilical pain, vomiting, and obstipation—the inability to pass gas or stool. Obstruction high in the small intestine is accompanied by vomiting.

251. The answer is b. *(Stobo, 23/e, pp 452–457.)* Localized epigastric burning pain relieved by eating requires evaluation for peptic ulcer disease. Upper gastrointestinal duodenoscopy provides the best sensitivity and specificity; barium swallow is less expensive, but is less sensitive and less accurate in defining mucosal disease. Patients with refractory or recurrent disease should have serum gastrin levels measured to rule out gastrinoma. A positive test for *H. pylori* would only indicate previous exposure.

252. The answer is c. *(Stobo, 23/e, p 452.)* Almost all patients with duodenal ulcer disease who are not on nonsteroidal anti-inflammatory agents are colonized with *H. pylori*. If *H. pylori* is eliminated, ulcers do not recur.

253. The answer is c. *(Stobo, 23/e, pp 454–455.) H. pylori* is not effectively treated by any single drug regimen. A two-week course of ampicillin, metronidazole, and bismuth is over 90% effective. Other regimens such as omperazole plus clarithromycin have also been successful. Patients with recurrent disease require *H. pylori* eradication; treatment of the first episode is more controversial.

254. The answer is c. *(Stobo, 23/e, pp 507–515.)* The first step in evaluating this patient with asymptomatic jaundice is to determine whether the increased bilirubin, as evidenced by scleral icterus, is conjugated or unconjugated hyperbilirubinemia. Patients with unconjugated hyperbilirubinemia do not have bilirubin in their urine because unconjugated bilirubin bound to albumin is not excreted in the urine.

255. The answer is a. *(Stobo, 23/e, pp 507–515.)* The patient has a conjugated hyperbilirubinemia with a cholestatic pattern of liver function tests. Normal enzymes rule out a disease-causing hepatocellular damage (such as viral or alcohol hepatitis). Instead, a disease of bile ducts or a cause of impaired bile excretion should be considered. Ultrasound or CT scan will evaluate the patient for biliary or pancreatic cancer or stone disease versus intrahepatic cholestasis.

256. The answer is a. *(Stobo, 23/e, pp 533–538.)* A paracentesis is required to evaluate new onset ascites. While cirrhosis and portal hypertension are most likely in this patient, complicating diseases such as tuberculous peritonitis and hepatoma are ruled out by analysis of ascitic fluid. An ultrasound or CT scan can be used to demonstrate ascitic fluid in equivocal cases.

257. The answer is a. *(Stobo, 23/e, pp 533–538.)* A serum albumin minus ascitic fluid albumin greater than 1.1 suggests portal hypertension alone as a cause for ascites. Tuberculous, pancreatitis, and malignancy should result in a difference of less than 1.1.

258. The answer is d. *(Stobo, 23/e, pp 537–538.)* Hepatic encephalopathy presents as a change of consciousness, behavior, and neuromuscular function associated with liver disease. Hyperreflexia and asterixis (the flapping tremor) are clinical manifestations of the disease process that results from toxins in the systemic circulation as a result of impaired hepatic clearance.

Fever, gastrointestinal bleeding, and sedation are all potential precipitating factors in a patient with liver disease. Hence, the patient described presents with typical signs and symptoms of hepatic encephalopathy. Meningitis, subdural hematoma, and postictal state all occur in the alcohol patient as well, and these may need to be distinguished from encephalopathy by additional tests such as lumbar puncture, CT scan, and EEG.

259. The answer is b. *(Stobo, 23/e, pp 430–438.)* The most likely diagnosis in this patient is esophageal carcinoma. Dysphagia is progressive first for solids and then liquids. There is blood in the stool and a history of weight loss. The patient has alcohol use and cigarette smoking as risk factors. Prognosis is not good, as once there is trouble swallowing, there is significant esophageal narrowing and the disease is usually incurable. A barium contrast study should demonstrate an esophageal carcinoma with marked narrowing and on irregular, ragged mucosal pattern. Ninety percent of esophageal carcinoma is squamous cell; 10% is adenocarcinoma. Achalasia should not cause guaiac-positive stools or progressive symptoms.

260. The answer is a. *(Stobo, 23/e, p 475.)* Microscopic examination of stool for leukocytes can help distinguish inflammatory from noninflammatory diarrhea. Only some infectious diarrheas are characterized by polymorphonuclear leukocytes. Leukocytes are common in *Shigella* diarrhea, but rare in rotavirus or Norwalk agent infection. *Entamoeba histolytica* can cause bloody diarrhea, but rarely produces many leukocytes.

261. The answer is c. *(Fauci, 14/e, pp 1704–1710.)* The patient's signs and symptoms suggest alcoholic hepatitis. Mallory bodies are alcoholic hyaline seen in damaged hepatocytes. Mallory bodies are likely to be seen in alcoholic hepatitis (but are not specific for the disease). Jugular venous distention should not be part of the process of chronic liver disease (ascites and pedal edema are secondary to hypoalbuminemia and portal hypertension, not increased right-sided pressure). In alcoholic hepatitis, AST-to-ALT ratios are usually greater than 2, due to the proportionately greater inhibition of ALT synthesis by ethanol. Even after abstinence, clinical recovery is often prolonged.

262. The answer is b. *(Fauci, 14/e, pp 1677–1691.)* The current hepatitis B vaccine is genetically engineered to consist of hepatitis B surface antigen particles. Therefore, only antibody to surface antigen will be detected after vaccination. Since the patient has had no exposure to hepatitis B, she should be surface antigen–negative.

263–265. The answers are 263-a, 264c, 265-b. *(Fauci, 14/e, pp 1649, 1707–1709, 1736.)* Primary biliary cirrhosis usually occurs in women between the ages of 35 and 60. The earliest symptom is pruritus, often accompanied by fatigue. Serum alkaline phosphatase is elevated two- to fivefold, and a positive antimitochondrial antibody test greater than 1:40 is both sensitive and specific.

Diverticulitis predisposes to liver abscess, particularly in the elderly patient. Liver abscess should be suspected in any patient with a history of abdominal infection who develops jaundice and right upper quadrant pain.

Obstructive jaundice that occurs in the setting of ulcerative colitis might be caused by gallstones or sclerosing cholangitis. Sclerosing cholangitis is a disorder characterized by a progressive inflammatory process of bile ducts. The diagnosis is usually made by demonstrating thickened ducts with narrow beaded lumina on cholangiography.

266. The answer is d. *(Fauci, 14/e, pp 1613–1615.)* A young man with recurrent ulcer disease unresponsive to therapy should be evaluated for Zollinger-Ellison syndrome—gastrin-containing tumors that are usually in the pancreas. The patient's serum gastrin level is elevated, but not diagnostic for gastrinoma (>1000 pg/ml). A secretin injection induces marked increases in gastrin levels in all patients with gastrinoma.

267. The answer is d. *(Fauci, 14/e, pp 2150–2151.)* Hemochromatosis is a disorder of iron storage that results in deposition of iron in parenchymal cells. The liver is usually enlarged, and excessive skin pigmentation is present in 90% of symptomatic patients at the time of diagnosis. Diabetes occurs secondary to direct damage of the pancreas by iron deposition. Arthropathy develops in 25 to 50% of cases. Other diagnoses listed could not explain all the manifestations of this patient's disease process.

268–270. The answers are 268-a, 269-b, 270-c. *(Fauci, 14/e, pp 1660–1667.)* The young black male with mild jaundice has an unconjugated hyperbilirubinemia and an anemia. This may be secondary to G6PD deficiency and an offending antibiotic (sulfonamide or trimethoprim-sulfamethoxazole). These patients are unable to maintain an adequate level of reduced glutathione in their red blood cells when antibiotic or other toxin causes increased metabolism of glucose.

The 60-year-old male with jaundice has an obstructive process, as his pale stools suggest the lack of bilirubin in the stool. A high-alkaline phosphatase also indicates that there is an obstructive jaundice. Pancreatic carcinoma would be the most likely cause of obstructive jaundice in this patient. The young woman's case is most consistent with acute hepatitis—very elevated hepatic enzymes and a conjugated hyperbilirubinemia.

271. The answer is a. *(Fauci, 14/e, pp 1677–1692.)* HBsAg appears in the circulation a few weeks before the onset of symptoms or abnormalities of serum biochemical parameters of liver function from acute hepatitis B infection. This antigen persists for a variable period during the acute illness and is usually cleared following formation of immune aggregates of HBsAg with HBsAb (the specific antibody). About 5 to 10% of patients do not develop surface antibody and fail to clear surface antigen. These patients are chronic carriers of hepatitis B and can develop chronic persistent hepatitis or chronic active hepatitis (serological pattern of choice A).

HBcAb develops during acute infection at about the time that serum aminotransferase (AST, ALT) levels become elevated. It usually persists for years. HBcAb is not a neutralizing antibody, and detection of this antibody does not signal recovery from hepatitis B infection. HBcAb is useful to diagnose acute infection during the window period—after surface antigen has disappeared and before surface antibody has appeared (serological pattern of choice B).

HBeAg is a marker for active viral replication and infectivity. It is useful in assessing the risk of viral transmission from an accidental needle stick (serological pattern of choice C).

HBsAb is usually detected during the late convalescent phase, four or more months after the onset of acute illness and weeks to months after the disappearance of surface antigen. HBsAb is a neutralizing and protective antibody. Development of this antibody signals recovery from acute infection and immunity from reinfection (serological pattern of choices D and E).

272. The answer is a. *(Fauci, 14/e, pp 1748–1751.)* Chronic pancreatitis is due to pancreatic damage from recurrent attacks of acute pancreatitis.

Insulin deficiency may result in diabetes mellitus. Vitamins D and K are absorbed intact from the intestines without digestion by lipase and are therefore absorbed normally in pancreatic insufficiency. Courvoisier's sign is a palpable, nontender gallbladder in a jaundiced patient. This finding suggests the presence of a malignancy, especially pancreatic cancer. Chronic pancreatitis per se does not produce guaiac-positive stools.

273. The answer is a. *(Bartlett, Rev Infect Dis 12 (suppl 2):243–251, 1990.)* *Clostridium difficile* is an important cause of diarrhea in patients who receive antibiotic therapy. *Clostridium difficile* proliferates in the gastrointestinal tract when the normal enteric flora is altered by antibiotics. Commonly implicated antibiotics include ampicillin, penicillin, clindamycin, cephalosporins, and trimethoprim-sulfamethoxazole. The diarrhea is usually mild to moderate, but can occasionally be profound. Other clinical findings include pyrexia, abdominal pain, abdominal tenderness, leukocytosis, and serum electrolyte abnormalities. The diagnosis is made by demonstration at sigmoidoscopy of yellowish plaques of pseudomembranes that cover the colonic mucosa or by detection of *Clostridium difficile* toxin in the stool. The pseudomembranes consist of a tenacious fibrinopurulent mucosal exudate that contains extruded leukocytes, mucin, and sloughed mucosa. Isolation of *Clostridium difficile* from stool cultures is not very specific because of asymptomatic carriage, particularly in infants. Serological tests are not clinically useful for diagnosing this infection. Pseudomembranous colitis demands discontinuance of the offending antibiotic. Antibiotic therapy for moderate or severe disease includes oral vancomycin or metronidazole. Cholestyramine and colestipol are also used therapeutically to bind the diarrheogenic toxin.

274–277. The answers are 274-e, 275-a, 276-b, 277-c. *(Fauci, 14/e, pp 1217–1222, 1717–1720.)* Alcoholic hepatitis typically presents with fever, pain, and tenderness of the right upper quadrant accompanied by hepatomegaly in an alcoholic patient. Typically the SGOT (serum glutamic-oxaloacetic transaminase, AST) level is much higher than the SGPT (serum glutamic-pyruvic transaminase, ALT) level. Although the diagnosis is usually made from these clinical findings, a liver biopsy would show prominent steatosis, or fat.

The blood fluke *Schistosoma mansoni* invades the portal vessels, where it stimulates intense inflammation and fibrosis. The portal vessels become pipelike, hence the name *pipestem fibrosis.* Schistosomiasis tends to produce portal hypertension with little derangement of liver function. Primary biliary cirrhosis is a disease of unknown etiology primarily affecting females. The inflammatory destruction in this disease of small- and medium-sized bile ducts eventually produces a paucity of bile ducts in the late stage of the disease.

Alpha$_1$-antitrypsin disease is a genetic disease in which the normal trypsin inhibitor alpha$_1$ antitrypsin is not produced. Symptoms are produced by hepatic or pulmonic injury. The diagnosis is supported by an absence of the normal spike produced by alpha$_1$ globulins on serum protein electrophoresis. For a definitive diagnosis, the serum alpha$_1$ antitrypsin form is determined by electrophoresis or by monoclonal antibodies. Liver biopsy characteristically demonstrates intracellular granules that are stained by the periodic acid Schiff's reagent and resist digestion with diastase.

278–281. The answers are 278-c, 279-d, 280-e, 281-b. *(Fauci, 14/e, pp 1702, 1719, 2150, 2166.)* Autoimmune hepatitis was formerly called *lupoid hepatitis* because it shares some features with systemic lupus erythematosus (SLE), such as the presence of an elevated titer of serum antinuclear antibodies (ANAs). This disease is treated by corticosteroids to reduce the immune-mediated hepatic injury. Type 1 disease occurs in young women who usually have marked hypergammaglobulinemia. (Type 2 disease occurs in children and is associated with a anti-LKM antibody.)

Wilson's disease is a hereditary disease of copper metabolism manifested by pathological deposition of copper in the liver, cornea, and brain. The serum ceruloplasmin level is almost always decreased with this disease. Another screening test is a slit-lamp ophthalmologic examination to detect the brown deposition on Descemet's membrane of the cornea, the Kayser-Fleischer rings.

Hemochromatosis is an autosomal recessive genetic disease of iron metabolism characterized by excessive iron absorption and abnormal iron storage within parenchymal organs, including the liver, pancreas, and heart. Hepatic deposition produces cirrhosis. With this disease, the serum ferritin level and the percentage of iron saturation (serum iron level divided by the total iron-building capacity, expressed as a percentage) are abnormally elevated because of excessive bodily iron. This disease is usually diagnosed by a liver biopsy.

Primary biliary cirrhosis is an idiopathic hepatic disease that primarily affects small- or medium-size bile ducts. It typically occurs in middle-aged females. Laboratory abnormalities include elevated serum alkaline phosphatase and bilirubin levels. Serum immunoelectrophoresis may demonstrate an elevated serum immunoglobulin M (IgM) level. Patients characteristically develop antimitochondrial antibodies.

282–285. The answers are 282-c, 283-a, 284-e, 285-a. *(Fauci, 14/e, pp 1707–1709, 2150–2151, 2168.)* Primary biliary cirrhosis is a disease of unknown etiology that primarily affects middle-aged women. Impaired biliary excretion of cholesterol due to progressive bile duct damage leads to hypercholesterolemia and to cholesterol deposition as xanthelasma on the eyelids and xanthomas on the arms.

Excessive copper deposition leads to disease of the liver and basal ganglia in Wilson's disease. Ocular findings include the premature development of large cataracts, called *sunflower cataracts,* and deposition of a brown pigment in Descemet's membrane of the cornea, a phenomenon called *Kayser-Fleischer rings.* Hemochromatosis is an inherited disease characterized by abnormally high iron absorption. Excessive iron is stored in the liver, pancreas, and heart. Subcutaneous iron deposition leads to bronzing of the skin.

NEPHROLOGY

DIRECTIONS: Each item below contains a question or incomplete statement followed by suggested responses. Select the **one best** response to each question.

Items 286–289

286. A 70-year-old male with a history of urinary tract infection and congestive heart failure was admitted to the hospital for sepsis and pulmonary edema. He was treated with clindamycin and tobramycin and also received intravenous furosemide. After several days, the signs of sepsis improved, but the BUN rose to 60 mg/dL and the creatinine to 5.0 mg/dL. The blood pressure was stable at 120/70, pulse 70, and there were no postural changes. Weight was unchanged throughout the hospital course. The most likely cause of the patient's deteriorating renal function is

a. Prerenal azotemia
b. Acute tubular necrosis
c. Interstitial nephritis
d. Hypercalcemic nephropathy

287. The best additional treatment for the above patient with acute renal failure, hyperkalemia, and ECG changes would include

a. Calcium gluconate
b. Polystyrene sulfonate
c. Bicarbonate
d. Low-potassium diet

288. The best evidence to support the diagnosis of acute tubular necrosis in this patient would be

a. Urine Na^+ of 25 meq/L
b. Renal tubular epithelial cells and muddy brown casts in urine sediment
c. A negative renal ultrasound
d. An intravenous pyelogram showing abnormalities of the medulla

289. Under what circumstances would this patient require acute hemodialysis?

a. BUN and creatinine do not return to normal after three days
b. The patient produces less than 200 cc of urine a day following the development of ATN
c. The patient develops hyperkalemia with peaked T waves and widening of the QRS complex
d. Urine sodium is more than 40 meq/liter

290. A 60-year-old male with a history of transient ischemic attacks had a cerebral angiogram one week ago. He presents with nausea and weakness and has a diffuse rash on exam. BP is 170/120 without postural changes. BUN is 90 meq/mL, and creatinine is 9 mg/dL. Urine sodium is greater than 40 meq/dl. Urine sediment is unremarkable. The most likely cause of this patient's renal failure is

a. Prerenal azotemia
b. Urinary tract obstruction
c. Atheroembolism
d. Interstitial nephritis

Items 291–292

291. A 70-year-old is found to be hypotensive in his home. He appears volume-depleted. Initial blood gases show a pH of 7.2, P_{CO_2} (mm Hg) 35. Other electrolytes are

Na^+ 136 meq/L	Cl^- 114
K^+ 4.0	HCO_3 14

The primary acid-base disorder in this patient is

a. Respiratory acidosis
b. Metabolic acidosis
c. Respiratory alkalosis
d. Metabolic alkalosis with compensation

292. The most likely cause of this acid-base disorder is

a. Renal failure
b. Diarrhea
c. Diabetic ketoacidosis
d. Alcohol ketoacidosis

293. A 25-year-old diabetic male is brought to the emergency room in coma with BP of 140/70 and P of 90. Blood sugar measurement by finger stick is elevated to 400. Blood gases show a pH of 7.2, HCO_3^- of 8 meq/L, P_{CO_2} of 33, BUN of 12 mg/dL, creatinine of 1.2 mg/dL. Anion gap is 18. The most likely cause of this metabolic acidosis is

a. Lactic acid
b. Acetoacetate and betahydroxybutyrate
c. Bicarbonate loss
d. Retained sulfate and phosphate anions

294. A young man presents to the emergency room with cyanosis and disorientation. Blood gases show a pH of 7.2, P_{CO_2} of 68 mm Hg, HCO_3^- of 25 meq/L. There are multiple needle tracks in the antecubital fossa. The rest of the examination is normal. The most likely acid-base problem is

a. Acute respiratory acidosis
b. Acute metabolic acidosis
c. Chronic respiratory acidosis
d. Chronic metabolic alkalosis with respiratory compensation

295. A 30-year-old female on birth control pills is seen in the emergency room with tachyphemia. She complains of parathesias. The pH is 7.5, HCO_3^- is 19 meq/L, P_{CO_2} is 25 mm Hg. Which of the following is correct?

a. The patient is having an anxiety attack
b. The most likely diagnosis is pulmonary embolus
c. The acid-base disorder is an acute respiratory alkalosis
d. The most likely cause of the alkalosis is vomiting

296. A 60-year-old male with severe chronic obstructive lung disease was admitted for respiratory failure with a pH of 7.3, HCO_3 of 40 meq/L, P_{CO_2} of 80 mm Hg. The patient required intubation and mechanical ventilation. On the ventilator his P_{CO_2} is now 40 mm Hg. The acid-base disorder that this patient is most likely to have is

a. Mild respiratory acidosis
b. Metabolic acidosis secondary to lactate
c. Metabolic alkalosis
d. There is not likely to be an acid-base disorder

297. A 65-year-old male with severe chronic bronchitis and CO_2 retention develops acute pneumococcal pneumonia and sepsis. Blood gases on admission show a pH of 7.0, P_{CO_2} of 65 mm Hg, HCO_3 of 8 meq/L. Serum Na^+ is 135, K^+ is 4.0, Cl is 110. The acid-base disorder is best described as

a. Pure respiratory acidosis
b. Mixed metabolic and respiratory acidosis
c. Pure metabolic acidosis
d. Mixed respiratory acidosis and metabolic alkalosis

Items 298–299

298. A 30-year-old male with HIV disease presents with complaints of flank pain and hematuria that have occurred suddenly. The patient, while being examined, is writhing in pain. A urinalysis shows many red blood cells without casts, few white blood cells. The most likely diagnosis in this patient is

a. Urolithiasis
b. Streptococcal glomerulonephritis
c. Bladder tumor
d. Pyelonephritis

299. The most important information in determining *the cause* of the stone in this patient is

a. The patient has had normal serum calcium determinations
b. The patient is taking Indinavir
c. The patient drinks two glasses of milk per day
d. The patient has been afebrile

300. A 40-year-old female with a history of Crohn's disease is s/p ileal resection when she develops flank pain and hematuria. One additional abnormality likely to be found in this patient is

a. Urine uric acid > 750 mg in 24 hours
b. Urine oxalate > 50 mg per 24 hours
c. Stag-horn calculi on KUB
d. Unexplained hypercalcemia

Items 301–302

301. A 60-year-old male with a history of small cell carcinoma of the lung is evaluated for fatigue and inability to concentrate. There is no history of polydipsia. His serum Na^+ is 125 meq/L. The patient's blood pressure is 130/80 sitting and standing, with a pulse of 80. There is no peripheral edema. Serum glucose and triglyceride levels are normal. Urine osmolality is 350 mmol/kg. BUN is 15 mg/dL, and creatinine is 1.0 mg/dL. This patient's hyponatremia is most likely explained by

a. Addison's disease
b. Edematous state
c. Recent diuretic therapy
d. Primary polydipsia
e. Ectopic vasopressin production

302. Treatment of choice for the above patient would be

a. Diuresis
b. Restriction of fluid
c. Lithium salts
d. Hypertonic saline

303. A 50-year-old male cigarette smoker works as a dry cleaner. He presents with a chief complaint of gross hematuria. There is no dysuria or flank pain. Urinalysis shows red blood cells without casts or white blood cells. The cause of the hematuria is most likely to be determined by

a. Intravenous pyelogram
b. Urine culture
c. Cystoscopy
d. Transrectal ultrasonography

304. A 40-year-old male was treated with clindamycin and gentamicin for acute diverticulitis. He has developed oliguria and an increasing serum creatinine over the past several days. On physical exam he is alert and oriented. There is no evidence for congestive heart failure. A three-component coarse heart sound is heard through systole and diastole. On the fifth hospital day, the BUN is 70 mg/dL, creatinine is 7 mg/dL, and serum K^+ is 5.0 meq/dL. An ECG shows acute ST-segment elevation in most leads. The next step in management would be

a. Acute hemodialysis
b. Pericardiocentesis
c. Thrombolytic therapy
d. Calcium gluconate
e. Aspirin 325 mg

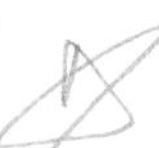

305. A 40-year-old woman with lymphoma has been receiving chemotherapy. Acute renal failure has developed with oliguria and a rapidly rising serum creatinine. Urinalysis shows red blood cells and many crystals. There are no muddy brown casts or renal tubular epithelial cells. There is no evidence for volume depletion on physical exam. A Foley catheter is placed, but there is only 100 cc of residual urine. The laboratory test most likely to yield a diagnosis is

a. Urine sodium
b. Serum uric acid
c. Serum calcium
d. Blood cultures

306. A 30-year-old man is transferred to the medical service five days after undergoing splenectomy for trauma. His blood urea nitrogen has risen to 100 mg/dL and his creatinine to 10 mg/dL. On exam there is normal skin turgor, chest is clear to auscultation and percussion, and there is no peripheral or sacral edema. The bladder is not distended by percussion. The most important information about this patient will come from

a. Renal biopsy
b. 24-hour urine protein
c. Urine sediment and spot urine sodium
d. Antinuclear antibody and serum complement

307. You are asked to evaluate a patient in the emergency room. He was brought by the rescue squad in a comatose state. Serum electrolytes drawn on admission show the following: Na^+ 133 meq/L, K^+ 8.0 meq/L, Cl of 98 meq/L, HCO_3 of 13 meq/L. An electrocardiogram shows a rhythm with absence of P waves, a widened QRS complex, and peaked T waves. Which would be the most appropriate initial step?

a. Repeat electrolyte measurements and observe
b. Attempt cardioversion
c. Administer intravenous calcium gluconate
d. Administer hydrochlorothiazide, 25 mg orally
e. Administer intravenous potassium chloride, 20 meq over 1 h

DIRECTIONS: Each group of questions below consists of lettered headings followed by a set of numbered items. For each numbered item select the **one** lettered heading with which it is most closely associated. Each lettered heading may be used once, more than once, or not at all.

Items 308–310

Match the clinical description with the most likely renal disease.

a. Hepatorenal syndrome
b. Acute tubular necrosis
c. Interstitial nephritis
d. Prerenal azotemia
e. Polycystic kidney disease
f. Acute obstruction
g. Poststreptococcal glomerulonephritis

308. A 30-year-old female complains of nausea and vomiting with associated diarrhea. Urine sodium is 8 meq/L. Urine specific gravity is 1.03.

309. Elderly male who has been recently hospitalized for confusion and treated with thorazine. Complains of mild lower abdominal pain. Has voided only 200 cc in 24 hours.

310. Hospitalized elderly woman is treated for gram-negative sepsis with ticarcillin and tobramycin. BUN is 80 meq/L. Creatinine is 8 meq/L. Urine sodium is 45 meq/L.

Items 311–314

Match each patient with the most likely renal calculi.

a. Calcium oxalate stones
b. Struvite (triple-phosphate) stones
c. Cystine stones
d. Uric acid stones

311. Patient with a myeloproliferative disorder

312. Patient with Crohn's disease

313. Patient with recurrent urinary tract infections by *Proteus* species

314. A 20-year-old man with recurrent stones; urinalysis shows many hexagonal crystals

Items 315–317.

Match the diuretic with the physiological properties noted below.

a. Increases reabsorption of calcium
b. Inhibits the $Na^+/K^+/2C^-$ carrier along the thick ascending loop of Henle
c. May induce a metabolic acidosis
d. Commonly causes hyperkalemia

315. Furosemide

316. Acetazolamide

317. Hydrochlorothiazide

Items 318–321

Match the drugs below with their characteristic nephrotoxic effect.

a. Allergic interstitial nephritis (AIN)
b. Nonoliguric acute tubular necrosis (ATN)
c. Crystalline nephropathy
d. Worsening azotemia in a patient with underlying renal insufficiency
e. Distal renal tubular acidosis

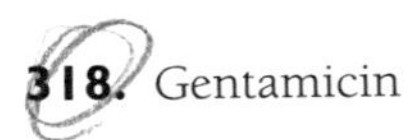

318. Gentamicin

319. Methicillin

320. Acyclovir

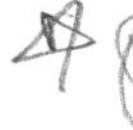

321. Tetracycline

NEPHROLOGY

Answers

286. The answer is b. *(Stobo, 23/e, pp 383–388.)* Since there is no clinical evidence of prerenal azotemia, it is most likely that this patient's acute renal failure is secondary to aminoglycoside toxicity and acute tubular necrosis.

287. The answer is a. *(Stobo, 23/e, p 386.)* When cardiac complications of severe hyperkalemia require emergency measures, the first line of therapy is intravenous calcium. Calcium increases the action potential, lessening the effect of membrane depolarization caused by hyperkalemia.

288. The answer is b. *(Stobo, 23/e, pp 383–388.)* The urine sediment in acute tubular necrosis is usually abnormal, with renal tubular epithelial cells, debris, and muddy brown casts. The high urine sodium, particularly if the patient has been getting a diuretic, is less specific. An ultrasound would rule out obstruction as a cause of renal failure, but would not be helpful in distinguishing prerenal from intrinsic renal failure. An IVP is contraindicated in the setting of acute renal failure.

289. The answer is c. *(Stobo, 23/e, pp 383–388.)* Hyperkalemia with cardiotoxicity is an indication for acute hemodialysis. The BUN and creatinine would not be expected to return to normal within days, and the patient may remain oliguric for several days or longer. The urine sodium is not a measure of recovery in ATN.

290. The answer is c. *(Fauci, 14/e, p 1309.)* Atheroembolism of the renal parenchyma occurs after angiographic exploration. Atheroma or cholesteral crystals are trapped within glomeruli. Emboli to the skin cause a livedo reticularis, usually over the abdomen and lower extemities. Retinal plaques may also be present.

291. The answer is b. *(Stobo, 23/e, p 377.)* The pH of 7.2 shows this to be a severe acidosis. The P_{CO_2} is less than 40 mm Hg; hence there is no CO_2 retention to suggest respiratory acidosis. The patient has a metabolic acidosis.

292. The answer is b. *(Stobo, 23/e, p 376.)* The anion gap is calculated to be 12. This is a normal anion gap (12 to 18). The patient therefore has a non–anion gap acidosis. Only diarrhea that causes bicarbonate loss will result in a non–anion gap acidosis. The other metabolic acidoses listed result in unmeasured anions and cause anion gap acidosis.

293. The answer is b. *(Stobo, 23/e, pp 377–381.)* The patient has a metabolic acidosis with an anion gap. Since he is a diabetic with an elevated blood sugar, diabetic ketoacidosis is the most likely cause for this anion gap acidosis. Retained anions are acetoacetate and betahydroxybutyrate. Some lactic acid accumulation is also possible, but the patient's blood pressure is stable, and this process would be much less likely. Since the patient is not in renal failure, retained sulfate and phosphate anions should not be responsible for the metabolic acidosis in this patient. There is no evidence given for bicarbonate loss—such as would occur with diarrhea.

294. The answer is a. *(Stobo, 23/e, p 379.)* The patient has an acidosis with a markedly elevated P_{CO_2}. The patient's cyanosis suggests hypoxia secondary to hypoventilation. The HCO_3^- is within normal range, suggesting that the respiratory acidosis is an acute process with no renal compensatory mechanism.

295. The answer is c. *(Stobo, 23/e, pp 380–381.)* The patient has an alkalosis with a very low P_{CO_2}—a respiratory alkalosis. Vomiting is a cause for metabolic alkalosis, which is not relevant here. Since information about the patient's oxygenation is not provided, one could not definitively distinguish between PE and panic attack. Both would cause acute hyperventilation and respiratory alkalosis.

296. The answer is c. *(Stobo, 23/e, pp 371–381.)* Prior to intubation, the patient had a chronic respiratory acidosis with a compensatory metabolic alkalosis. Once ventilated, the respiratory acidosis resolved, leaving what would certainly be a significant metabolic alkalosis.

297. The answer is b. *(Stobo, 23/e, pp 377–381.)* The patient has a severe acidosis, with both an elevated P_{CO_2} and a very low bicarbonate. This is caused by hypoventilation and sepsis. The patient is most likely to have a lactic acidosis associated with the infectious process. It is an anion gap acidosis.

298. The answer is a. *(Stobo, 23/e, pp 413–417.)* The patient presents with clinical features of a renal stone, which is supported by the findings of red blood cells in the urine sediment. Red blood cell casts would be expected in glomerular disease, white blood cells in pyelonephritis. The patient's symptoms are not consistent with bladder cancer.

299. The answer is b. *(Fauci, 14/e, p 1850; Stobo, 23/e, pp 413–417.)* Indinavir causes urolithiasis in about 4% of patients. Patients on this medication must maintain excellent fluid intake. These stones are the result of precipitation of crystals of the drug itself. Patients with calcium-containing stones usually have normal serum calcium levels and do not have increased levels of dietary calcium. There is an abnormally high absorption of calcium in many patients. The presence or absence of fever is not helpful in determining the etiology of renal stones. However, patients with chronic urinary tract infection, particularly with urea-splitting organisms such as *Proteus* species, are more likely to have struvite stones, a complex of magnesium—ammonium phosphate and carbonate apatite.

300. The answer is b. *(Stobo, 23/e, pp 413–417.)* Patients with Crohn's disease and ileal resection have fat malabsorption. Calcium in the bowel lumen is bound by fatty acids instead of oxalate. Oxalate is then left free for absorption in the colon. Increased oxalate absorption can result in oxalate stone production.

301. The answer is e. *(Stein, 5/e, pp 812–814.)* The patient has hyponatremia without evidence of edema or volume depletion. The urine osmolality is high, greater than 300 mmol/kg. The patient has small cell carcinoma, which is the most common tumor to produce ectopic antidiuretic hormone. All of these clues suggest inappropriate ADH secretion. Adrenocortical insufficiency would be unlikely without hypotension. Normal glucose and triglyceride levels rule out pseudohyponatremia.

302. The answer is b. *(Stein, 5/e, pp 812–814.)* Restriction of fluid to 800 to 1000 ml is the foundation of treatment for SIADH. A negative water balance will result in gradual increase in the serum sodium. Sodium chloride infusion is used cautiously and only when severe confusion, convulsions, or coma is evident. Lithium does interfere with the action of ADH on tubular water reabsorption, but it can cause serious side effects and is generally not recommended.

303. The answer is c. *(Stobo, 23/e, pp 793–794.)* The patient is at risk for bladder carcinoma both because of cigarette smoking and because of exposure to aromatic hydrocarbons as a dry cleaner. Gross hematuria is the most common first sign of bladder tumor. While gross hematuria from a renal stone, prostatic disease, or hypernephroma cannot be ruled out, bladder cancer is a more likely explanation for this clinical picture, and cystoscopy with urinary cytologic evaluation is the procedure most likely to provide definitive diagnosis.

304. The answer is a. *(Stein, 5/e, p 774.)* A pericardial rub that develops in the setting of acute renal failure is an indication for acute hemodialysis. A cardiac echo should be performed, but pericardiocentesis would not be indicated unless there was evidence for tamponade. Diffuse ST-segment elevations suggest pericarditis and not ischemia.

305. The answer is b. *(Stobo, 23/e, pp 235–236.)* The case is a classic picture of acute uric acid nephropathy. Acute overproduction of uric acid and extreme hyperuricemia lead to the rapid development of renal failure. The process is usually seen in patients with lymphoproliferative disease who have been given chemotherapy. Uric acid crystals are deposited in the kidneys and collecting system, leading to partial or complete obstruction. Uric acid crystals are found in the urine, and serum uric acid levels are very high, almost always above 20 mg/dL.

306. The answer is c. *(Fauci, 14/e, pp 1504–1512.)* The initial evaluation in this patient is aimed toward obtaining further information so that the cause of acute renal failure may be characterized as either prerenal, renal, or postrenal (obstruction). Of those tests listed, the urine sodium and urine sediment would be the most helpful. A urine sodium greater than 40 meq/L suggests that acute tubular necrosis is more likely than prerenal azotemia. A urine sediment that shows renal tubular epithelial cells and muddy brown casts is diagnostic for acute tubular necrosis.

307. The answer is c. *(Rose, 4/e, pp 845–852.)* This patient presents with severe hyperkalemia. Although potassium elevations can occasionally be spurious (e.g., in hemolysis), the changes on this patient's ECG reflect severe cardiotoxic effects from the hyperkalemia. The ECG shows a typical progression in hyperkalemia, with peaked T waves followed by widening of the QRS, loss of P waves, and eventually a sine wave pattern. Therapy of severe hyperkalemia includes intravenous calcium gluconate (to normalize membrane excitability), glucose and insulin, sodium bicarbonate (to drive potassium intracellularly), and potassium exchange resins (to remove potassium). Dialysis may be necessary, particularly in patients with concomitant renal failure.

308–310. The answers are 308-d, 309-f, 310-b. *(Fauci, 14/e, pp 1507–1513.)* The 30-year-old female patient has clinical symptoms that could result in volume depletion. The high specific gravity of the urine and high urine sodium make prerenal azotemia the most likely diagnosis. The elderly patient with oliguria and lower abdominal pain should be evaluated for urinary tract obstruction, a side effect of many psychotropic medications, particularly in older males with prostatic hypertrophy. The elderly female patient has developed acute tubular necrosis secondary to either hypotension or aminoglycoside therapy.

311–314. The answers are 311-d, 312-a, 313-b, 314-c. *(Fauci, 14/e, pp 1569–1574.)* Nephrolithiasis is becoming an increasingly prevalent problem in Western society. Patients with renal stones often present with signs of partial or complete obstruction, flank or abdominal pain, and hematuria. Calcium oxalate (alone or in combination with apatite) stones are by far the most common, accounting for approximately three-quarters of all stones. They are typically radiodense and therefore can often be detected on plain abdominal films. Hypercalciuria (with or without hypercalcemia), hyperoxaluria, hyperuricosuria, decreased urinary citrate, and decreased urine volumes can all predispose to calcium oxalate precipitation. Hyperoxaluria can be either primary (i.e., an inherited enzyme defect) or acquired. The most common cause of the latter is the increased intestinal absorption of oxalate in patients with small-intestinal bypass or inflammatory bowel disease (such as Crohn's disease).

Struvite (triple-phosphate) stones are most commonly seen in patients with recurrent infections with uricase-producing bacteria (such as *Proteus*). Urease-driven conversion of urea to ammonia and CO_2 (and eventually NH_4^+ and HCO_3^-) supports a persistently alkaline urine (pH greater than 7.5), which favors the formation of struvite ($MgNH_4PO_46H_2O$) crystals. These stones are also radiopaque, and occasionally they can become quite large within the renal pelvis and calyces (so-called stag-horn calculi).

Uric acid stones account for from 5 to 10% of all stones. In contrast to calcium oxalate and struvite, these stones are usually radiolucent. Hyperuricemia and attendant hyperuricosuria (such as is seen in myeloproliferative disorders or with defects of purine synthesis) can predispose to uric acid stones. Acid urine and low urine volumes also favor stone formation. Raising urine pH to above 6.0 to 6.5 can be very effective in solubilizing uric acid.

Cystine stones are relatively rare and occur in patients with an inherited disorder of amino acid handling that results in excessive urinary excretion of cystine, ornithine, lysine, and arginine. The urinalysis often shows the distinctive hexagon-shaped cystine crystals.

315–317. The answers are 315-b, 316-c, 317-a. *(Rose, 4/e, pp 426–432.)* Diuretics enhance salt excretion by inhibiting NaCl reabsorption at various tubular sites. Acetazolamide, by inhibiting carbonic anhydrase, decreases Na^+, Cl^-, and HCO_3^- reclamation along the proximal tubule. The ensuing loss of alkali (as $NaHCO_3$) can evoke a metabolic acidosis. Acetazolamide, however, is a relatively weak diuretic, partially because of the ability of more distal sites to increase solute reabsorption. The loop diuretics (furosemide, bumetanide, and ethacrynic acid) are the most potent diuretics. They inhibit the $Na^+/K^+/2Cl^-$ transporter along the loop of Henle. These agents also inhibit calcium reabsorption at this site and thereby increase calcium excretion.

The thiazide diuretics inhibit Na^+ and Cl^- reabsorption along the distal tubule (and connecting segment) and induce a modest natriuresis. Contrary to the loop diuretics, these agents increase calcium reabsorption, presumably both by a direct distal effect and at the proximal tubule (owing to volume depletion).

318–321. The answers are 318-b, 319-a, 320-c, 321-d. *(Fauci, 14/e, pp 1505–1513.)* Nephrotoxicity can be an important manifestation of drug toxicity, especially since many agents are primarily excreted through the kidneys. The nephrotoxicity of the aminoglycosides (including gentamicin) is well recognized and tends to occur in from 2 to 20% of patients treated. The patients typically present with nonoliguric renal failure (ATN) several days after initiation of therapy. Risk factors for aminoglycoside nephrotoxicity include increased age, preexisting renal disease, volume contraction, repeated doses, and the use of other nephrotoxic agents. Treatment is generally supportive, as the majority of patients will recover renal function after discontinuation of the drug. Rare patients with severe renal failure may require dialysis. Allergic interstitial nephritis (AIN) is another well-recognized drug effect. Many agents have been associated with AIN, including the penicillins (especially methicillin), cephalosporins, sulfa drugs, and diuretics. Characteristically, the patients present with rash, fever, azotemia, eosinophilia, and eosinophiluria. The kidneys may show increased gallium uptake and are typically enlarged. Usually, the renal function improves after the offending agent is stopped (though this may take several days). The role of steroids in the management of AIN remains controversial.

The antiviral agent acyclovir can be associated with acute crystalline nephropathy due to the limited solubility of the agent. It is essential that intravenous acyclovir be given slowly (over at least 60 min) to prevent this effect.

Owing to their decreased anabolism, the tetracyclines are often associated with worsening azotemia when given to patients with renal insufficiency. If a patient with renal failure requires a tetracycline, the preferred one is doxycycline because its ananabolic effect is the least pronounced. Outdated tetracycline has been associated with a proximal renal tubular acidosis, and demeclocycline (another tetracycline derivative) can cause polyuria by inducing a renal-concentrating defect.

HEMATOLOGY AND ONCOLOGY

DIRECTIONS: Each item below contains a question or incomplete statement followed by suggested responses. Select the **one best** response to each question.

322. A 55-year-old male is being evaluated for constipation and change in bowel habits. He has no history of gastrectomy or upper GI symptoms. Hemoglobin is 10 g/dL. Mean corpuscular volume (MCV) is 72 fl, serum iron 8 μmol/L (normal: 9 to 27), iron-binding capacity 75 μmol/L (normal: 45 to 66), saturation 10% (normal: 20 to 40%), ferritin 10 μg/L (normal: 15 to 400 μg/L). The next step in the evaluation of this patient's anemia would be

a. Red blood cell folate
b. Iron absorption studies
c. Sigmoidoscopy
d. Lead level

323. A 50-year-old woman has complained of pain and swelling in her proximal interphalangeal joints, both wrists and knees. She complains of morning stiffness. She has had a hysterectomy 10 years ago. Physical exam shows swelling and thickening of the PIP joints. Hemoglobin is 10.3 g/dL, MCV 80 fl, serum iron 8 μmol/L, iron-binding capacity 40 μmol/L (normal: 45 to 66), saturation 20%. The most likely explanation for this woman's anemia is

a. Occult blood loss
b. Vitamin deficiency
c. Anemia of chronic disease
d. Sideroblastic anemia

324. A 35-year-old female is recovering from *Mycoplasma pneumoniae* pneumonia and feels weak. Her Hgb is 9.0 g/dL with a normal MCV. The best test to determine whether the patient has a hemolytic anemia is

a. Serum bilirubin
b. Reticulocyte count and blood smear
c. Mycoplasma antigen
d. Serum LDH

Items 325–327

325. A 70-year-old male complains of two months of low back pain and fatigue. He has developed a fever with purulent sputum production. On physical exam he has pain over several vertebrae and rales at the left base. Laboratory results are as follows:

Hemoglobin	7 g/dL
MCV	86 fl (normal 86 to 98)
WBC	12,000 cu/mm
BUN	44 mg/dL
Creatinine	3.2 mg/dL
Ca^{++}	11.5 mg/dL
Chest x-ray	LLL infiltrate
Reticulocyte count	1%

The most likely diagnosis is

a. Multiple myeloma
b. Lymphoma
c. Metastatic bronchogenic carcinoma
d. Primary hyperparathyroidism

326. The definitive diagnosis is best made by

a. 24-hour urine protein
b. Greater than 10% plasma cells in bone marrow
c. Renal biopsy
d. Rouleaux formation on blood smear

327. Renal insufficiency may have developed in this patient secondary to

a. Collecting tubules obstructed by Bence Jones protein
b. Hypercalcemia
c. Amyloid deposition
d. Plasma cell infiltration of the kidney
e. All of the above

328. After undergoing surgical resection for carcinoma of the stomach, a 60-year-old male has developed numbness in his feet. On exam he has lost proprioception in the lower extremities and has a wide-based gait and positive Romberg. A peripheral blood smear shows macrocytosis and hypersegmented polymorphonuclear leukocytes. The neurologic dysfunction is secondary to

a. Folic acid
b. Thiamine
c. Vitamin K
d. Vitamin B_{12}

Items 329–330

329. A 60-year-old asymptomatic man was found to have a leukocytosis when a routine CBC was obtained. Physical exam shows no abnormalities. The spleen is of normal size. Lab data includes

Hgb	9 g/dL (normal: 14 to 18)
Leukocyte count	40,000/mm^3 (normal: 4300 to 10,800)

Peripheral blood smear shows a differential that includes 97% small lymphocytes. The most likely diagnosis is

a. Acute monocytic leukemia
b. Chronic myelogenous leukemia
c. Chronic lymphocyte leukemia
d. Tuberculosis

330. This patient would require chemotherapy

a. If the white blood cell count rises
b. If lymphadenopathy develops
c. To control anemia or thrombocytopenia
d. Only when acute lymphocytic leukemia develops

331. A 45-year-old male presents with pancytopenia and splenomegaly. There is no peripheral adenopathy. Peripheral blood smear shows white blood cells with long cytoplasmic projections. The treatment of choice is

a. Splenectomy
b. Cladribine, a purine analogue
c. Interferon alpha
d. Cytoxan

332. A 38-year-old female presents with recurrent sore throat. She is on no medications, does not use ethanol, and has no history of renal disease. Physical exam is normal. A CBC shows an Hgb of 9.0 mg/dL, white blood cell count of 2000 mm^3, and a platelet count of 30,000 mm^3. The best approach to diagnosis would be

a. Erythropoietin level
b. Serum B_{12}
c. Bone marrow biopsy
d. Liver spleen scan

Items 333–334

333. A 50-year-old female complains of vague abdominal pain, constipation, and a sense of fullness in the lower abdomen. On physical exam the abdomen is nontender, but there is shifting dullness to percussion. The next step in evaluation is

a. Abdominal ultrasound
b. Pelvic examination
c. CA 125 cancer antigen
d. Sigmoidoscopy

334. Risk factors for this malignancy include

a. Infertility
b. Oral contraceptives
c. Coitus early in life
d. Multiple partners

Items 335–360

335. A 40-year-old male complains of hematuria. He has a aching pain in his flank. Laboratory data show a normal BUN, creatinine, and electrolytes. Hemoglobin is elevated at 14 g/dL and serum calcium is 11 mg/dL. A solid renal mass is found by ultrasound. The most likely diagnosis is

a. Polycystic kidney disease
b. Renal carcinoma
c. Adrenal adenoma
d. Urolithiasis

336. The best choice for cure in this patient would be

a. Nephrectomy
b. Radiation therapy
c. Interferon alpha
d. Interleukin-2

337. A 20-year-old male finds a mass in his scrotum. The *first* step in evaluating this mass is

a. Palpation and transillumination
b. HCG and alpha fetoprotein
c. Scrotal ultrasonography
d. Evaluation for inguinal adenopathy

338. A 25-year-old had a splenectomy for traumatic injury. After the splenectomy, this patient had a normal CBC, except for a platelet count of 500,000 (normal: 130,000 to 400,000/mm^3). The best approach to evaluating this thrombocytosis is

a. Evaluate for infection
b. Evaluate for malignancy
c. Obtain bone marrow aspirate
d. Observe without workup

Items 339–340

339. A patient has been complaining of fatigue and night sweats associated with itching for two months. On physical exam there is diffuse nontender lymphadenopathy, including small supraclavicular, epitrochlear, and scalene nodes. A chest x-ray shows hilar lymphadenopathy. The next step in evaluation would be

a. Excisional lymph node biopsy
b. Monospot test
c. Toxoplasmosis IgG
d. Angiotensin converting enzyme

340. The patient described is found on biopsy to have mixed cellularity Hodgkin's lymphoma. Liver function tests are normal, and the spleen is nonpalpable. The next step in evaluation would be

a. CT scan or MRI
b. Liver biopsy
c. Repeat node biopsy
d. Erythrocyte sedimentation rate

Items 341–342

341. A 62-year-old black man presents with hypertension, a decreased urine stream, and low back pain. The physical examination shows a hard, nodular left prostatic lobe and percussion tenderness in the lumbar vertebral bodies and left seventh rib. The next step in evaluation would be

a. Bone scan
b. Biopsy of prostate
c. CT scan
d. Bone marrow biopsy

342. The patient is found to have adenocarcinoma of the prostate with bony metastases. Treatment of choice would be

a. Observation
b. Radiation therapy
c. Estrogen therapy
d. Flutamide and luteinizing hormone–releasing hormone (LHRH)
e. Chemotherapy

Items 343–344

343. A 68-year-old male is hospitalized with a transient ischemic attack and is evaluated for carotid disease. Physical exam is normal. A CBC on admission is normal. The patient is started on heparin. A repeat CBC one week later shows an Hgb of 14 g/dL (normal: 13 to 18), WBC of 9,000/mm^3, and platelet count of 10,000/mm^3. You would

a. Obtain bone marrow study
b. Obtain liver-spleen scan
c. Suspect drug-induced thrombocytopenia
d. Begin corticosteroids for idiopathic thrombocytopenia purpura

344. The patient described develops thrombosis of the brachial artery. The next step in management would be

a. Lupus anticoagulant
b. Antinuclear antibody
c. Stop heparin
d. Increase heparin dose

345. A patient with bacterial endocarditis develops thrombophlebitis while hospitalized. His course in the hospital is uncomplicated. On discharge he is treated with penicillin, rifampin, and Coumadin. Therapeutic prothrombin levels are obtained on 15 mg of Coumadin per day. After two weeks, the penicillin and rifampin are discontinued. You would now

a. Cautiously increase Coumadin dosage
b. Continue Coumadin at 15 mg/d for about six months
c. Reduce Coumadin dosage
d. Stop Coumadin therapy

346. A 65-year-old male with diabetes mellitus, bronzed skin, and cirrhosis of the liver is being treated for hemochromatosis previously confirmed by liver biopsy. The patient experiences increasing right upper quadrant pain, and his serum alkaline phosphatase is now elevated. There is a 15-pound weight loss. The next step in management would be

a. Increase frequency of phlebotomy for worsening hemochromatosis
b. Obtain CT scan to rule out hepatoma
c. Obtain hepatitis B serology
d. Obtain antimitochondrial antibody to rule out primary biliary cirrhosis

347. A 40-year-old cigarette smoker is found on routine physical exam to have a 1-cm white patch on his oral mucosa that does not rub off. There are no other lesions in the mouth. The patient has no risk factors for HIV infection. The lesion is nontender. The next step in management would be

a. Culture for *Candida albicans*
b. Follow lesion with annual physical exam
c. Biopsy lesion
d. Reassure patient that this is normal variant

DIRECTIONS: Each group of questions below consists of lettered headings followed by a set of numbered items. For each numbered item select the **one** lettered heading with which it is most closely associated. Each lettered heading may be used once, more than once, or not at all.

Items 348–352

Match the anticancer drug with its most likely toxicity.

a. Pulmonary fibrosis
b. Cardiotoxicity
c. Nephrotoxicity
d. Peripheral neuropathy
e. Vaginal bleeding
f. Steatorrhea
g. Intestinal ulcers
f. Angioedema

348. Cisplatin

349. Bleomycin

350. Doxorubicin

351. Vincristine

352. Tamoxifen

DIRECTIONS: Each item below contains a question or incomplete statement followed by suggested responses. Select the **one best** response to each question.

353. A 20-year-old black male with sickle cell anemia, SS homozygote, has had several episodes of painful crises. The least likely physical finding in this patient would be

a. Scleral icterus
b. Systolic murmur
c. Splenomegaly
d. Ankle ulcers

354. A 30-year-old black man plans a trip to India and is advised to take prophylaxis for malaria. Three days after beginning treatment, he • develops dark urine, pallor, fatigue, and jaundice. Hematocrit is 30% (it had been 43%) and reticulocyte count is 7%. He stops taking the medication. Treatment should consist of

a. Splenectomy
b. Administration of methylene blue
c. Administration of vitamin E
d. Exchange transfusions
e. No additional treatment is required

Items 355–356

355. A 58-year-old Scandinavian male presents with shortness of breath and is found to have anemia. Peripheral blood smear shows macrocytosis and hypersegmented polyps. The patient also has postural hypotension. Skin shows both vitiligo and hyperpigmentation. Romberg sign is positive. Serum sodium is 120 meq/L (normal: 136 to 145) and potassium is 5.2 meq/L (normal: 3.5 to 5.0) Urinary sodium is increased. Which of the following is correct?

a. The patient's symptoms will be explained on the basis of folate deficiency
b. Only 50% of such patients will have parietal cell antibody
c. The patient is likely to have low levels of vitamin B_{12} and high levels of intrinsic factor
d. The patient is likely to have low levels of vitamin B_{12} and decreased secretion of intrinsic factor

356. In addition to anemia this patient is most likely to have

a. Addison's disease of autoimmune etiology
b. Pituitary insufficiency
c. Hemochromatosis
d. Inappropriate ADH secretion

357. A 70-year-old intensive care unit patient complains of fever and shaking chills. The patient develops hypotension, and blood cultures are positive for gram-negative bacilli. The patient begins bleeding from venipuncture sites and around his Foley catheter.

Hct: 38%
WBC: 15.00×10^3 mm
Platelet count: 40,000 per mm^3 (normal: 130,000 to 400,000)
Peripheral blood smear: fragmented RBCs
PT: elevated
PTT: elevated
Plasma fibrinogen: 70 mg/dL (200 to 400)

The best course of therapy in this patient is

a. Begin heparin
b. Treat underlying disease
c. Begin plasmapheresis
d. Give vitamin K
e. Begin red blood cell transfusion

358. A 30-year-old female with Graves' disease has been started on propylthiouracil. She complains of low-grade fever, chills, and sore throat. The most important initial step in evaluating this patient's fever is

a. Serum TSH
b. Serum T_3
c. CBC
d. Chest x-ray
e. Blood cultures

DIRECTIONS: Each group of questions below consists of lettered headings followed by a set of numbered items. For each numbered item select the **one** lettered heading with which it is most closely associated. Each lettered heading may be used once, more than once, or not at all.

Items 359–361

Match the clinical description with the most likely diagnosis.

a. Sideroblastic anemia
b. Thalassemia
c. Iron-deficiency anemia
d. Anemia of renal disease
e. Lead poisoning

359. Alcoholic patient being treated for tuberculosis has increase in serum iron and transferrin saturation

360. Low serum iron, elevated iron-binding capacity of serum

361. Normocytic, normochromic anemia

Items 362–365

Match the description with the type of leukemia:

a. Chronic myelocytic leukemia
b. Acute myelocytic anemia
c. Acute lymphocytic leukemia
d. Chronic myelogenous leukemia
e. Acute premyelocytic leukemia
f. Hairy cell leukemia

362. Sticklike abnormal primary granules may be present in cytoplasm of leukemia cells.

363. Frequently associated with disseminated intravascular coagulation induced by thromboplastic material released by leukemic cells.

364. Pancytopenia, splenomegaly. Cytoplasmic projections may be seen on peripheral smear.

365. More than 90% of patients have leukemic cells with deoxynucleotidyl transferase.

HEMATOLOGY AND ONCOLOGY

Answers

322. The answer is c. *(Stobo, 23/e, pp 707–711.)* The patient has a microcytic anemia. A low serum iron, low ferritin, and high iron-binding capacity all are consistent with iron-deficiency anemia. Most iron-deficiency anemia is explained by blood loss. The patient's symptoms of constipation point to blood loss from the lower GI tract. Sigmoidoscopy would be the highest-yield procedure. Lead poisoning can cause a microcytic, hypochromic anemia, but this would be uncommon in a 55-year-old male with no clues to suggest the diagnosis. Folate deficiency presents as a megaloblastic anemia.

323. The answer is c. *(Fauci, 23/e, pp 643–644.)* The patient described has a hypoproliferative anemia, called an *inflammatory anemia* or *anemia of chronic disease*. It is characterized by a low serum iron and a low iron-binding capacity with a saturation of between 10 and 20%. The anemia is usually normocytic, normochromic, but may be mildly microcytic. The process occurs as a result of release of inflammatory cytokines, which cause a suppressive effect on erythropoiesis.

324. The answer is b. *(Fauci, 23/e, pp 669–671.)* An elevated reticulocyte count in a patient with normocytic, normochromic anemia strongly suggests hemolysis. The reticulocyte count must be corrected for degree of anemia. Peripheral blood smear may show abnormalities of shape that can suggest hemolysis. Indirect bilirubin and serum LDH are usually mildly elevated in hemolytic anemia, but are less specific.

325. The answer is a. *(Fauci, 14/e, pp 713–717.)* The onset of multiple myeloma is usually insidious, with weakness and fatigue. Pain caused by bone involvement, anemia, renal insufficiency, and bacterial pneumonia often follow. This patient presented with fatigue and bone pain and then developed bacterial pneumonia probably secondary to *S. pneumoniae*, an encapsulated organism for which antibody to the polysaccharide capsule is not adequately produced by the myeloma patient. There is also evidence for renal insufficiency. Hypercalcemia is frequently seen in patients with multiple myeloma and may be life-threatening.

326. The answer is b. *(Fauci, 14/e, pp 713–717.)* Definitive diagnosis is made by demonstrating greater than 10% plasma cells in bone marrow. None of the other findings are specific enough for definitive diagnosis. Renal biopsy would not be helpful.

327. The answer is e. *(Fauci, 14/e, pp 713–717.)* Renal insufficiency occurs in about half of all myeloma patients. All factors listed may play a role in real insufficiency. In addition, acute and chronic pyelonephritis also occurs. Acute renal failure can occur after intravenous urography, which should be avoided in the myeloma patient.

328. The answer is d. *(Fauci, 14/e, pp 653–659.)* These neurologic deficits occur with vitamin B_{12} deficiency. This patient has a deficit of intrinsic factor after gastric surgery. Folic acid deficiency causes a megaloblastic anemia, but not neurologic deficits.

329. The answer is c. *(Stobo, 23/e, p 744.)* Chronic lymphocytic leukemia is the most common of all leukemias, with an increasing incidence with age. Patients are usually asymptomatic, but may complain of weakness, fatigue, or enlarged lymph nodes. The diagnosis is made by peripheral blood smear, as mature small lymphocytes constitute almost all the white blood cells seen. No other process produces a lymphocytosis of this morphology and magnitude.

330. The answer is c. *(Stobo, 23/e, p 744.)* Indications for chemotherapy in CLL include control of anemia or thrombocytopenia. It may also be used to reduce bulky adenopathy or splenomegaly. Early treatment of this disease does not improve survival.

331. The answer is b. *(Stobo, 23/e, p 744.)* The disease described is hairy cell leukemia, which typically presents with leukopenia and splenomegaly. Infection, particularly Legionnaires' disease, complicates the course of the disease. The treatment of hairy cell leukemia has been revolutionized with cladribine, which induces a clinical remission in over 80% of patients.

Some remissions last for more than three years. Splenectomy and interferon alpha had been used prior to cladribine.

332. The answer is c. *(Stobo, 23/e, pp 701–706.)* This young woman has an unexplained pancytopenia. There is no drug history or toxin to explain this bone marrow effect. A bone marrow biopsy is the diagnostic method of choice.

333. The answer is b. *(Stobo, 23/e, pp 786–787.)* The first step in this patient's evaluation is a pelvic exam to rule out ovarian cancer. Pelvic fullness, vague discomfort, constipation, and early satiety are often the first symptoms of this process. Ascites may be present on initial evaluation. Abdominal ultrasound would follow. The CA 125 cancer antigen supports the diagnosis of ovarian cancer, but it is not sensitive or specific. If the pelvic exam and ultrasound were negative, sigmoidoscopy might be indicated to evaluate the patient's constipation.

334. The answer is a. *(Stobo, 23/e, pp 786–787.)* Infertility is a risk factor for ovarian cancer. Women treated for infertility for over one year appear to be at risk. Oral contraceptives may be somewhat protective. Coitus early in life and multiple partners are risk factors for cervical, but not ovarian, carcinoma.

335. The answer is b. *(Stobo, 23/e, p 792.)* Renal carcinoma tends to occur in males from 40 to 60 years of age. Hematuria, flank pain, and palpable abdominal mass are the triad of common symptoms. Paraneoplastic syndromes are common, including erythrocytosis and hypercalcemia.

336. The answer is a. *(Stobo, 23/e, p 792.)* Radical nephrectomy, including removal of the kidney, surrounding fascia, adrenal gland, and regional lymph nodes provides the only chance for cure in patients with renal cell carcinoma. Radiation therapy is used in metastatic renal carcinoma, but results are disappointing. Immunotherapy such as interferon and interleukin 2 have been used for palliation.

337. The answer is a. *(Stobo, 23/e, pp 794–796.)* The first step in evaluating a scrotal mass is to determine whether the mass is in the testis or outside the testis. Most solid masses rising from within the testis are malignant. Palpation of the scrotal mass and transillumination (holding a flashlight directly against the posterior wall of the scrotum) will distinguish testicular lesions from other masses within the scrotum, such as hydrocele. Ultrasonography will confirm a solid testicular mass. HCG and alpha fetoprotein are important in assessment of seminoma versus nonseminomatous testicular cancer, once testicular mass lesion is confirmed.

338. The answer is d. *(Fauci, 14/e, p 683.)* Platelet counts to this level occur after splenectomy. No further workup is indicated. The differential of thrombocytosis includes postsplenectomy platelet elevations.

339. The answer is a. *(Stobo, 23/e, pp 797–801.)* The long-term nature of these symptoms, the fact that the nodes are nontender, and their location, including scalene and supraclavicular, all suggest the likelihood of malignancy. Hence, toxoplasmosis and EBV virus are unlikely causes of this clinical picture. An angiotensin converting enzyme test would give nonspecific evidence for sarcoidosis, a possible diagnosis. Excisional biopsy is necessary to rule out malignancy, particularly lymphoma.

340. The answer is a. *(Stobo, 23/e, pp 797–801.)* The staging of Hodgkin's disease is important so that proper treatment can be determined. To determine whether the patient has stage III or IV disease, the presence or absence of disease in the abdomen must be known. A CT scan or an MRI of the abdomen would be the test of choice. Staging laparotomy is not as necessary as in the past because these imaging tests can usually identify or exclude disease of the abdomen.

341. The answer is b. *(Stobo, 23/e, pp 790–791.)* A prostatic biopsy is necessary to confirm the diagnosis of prostatic carcinoma. A metastatic workup, including bone scan, would then follow. Bone scan is routinely used to evaluate for metastatic disease. Imaging of pelvic nodes by CT is unreliable because of lack of sensitivity. CT is also unable to reliably detect spread of prostatic cancer beyond the capsule.

342. The answer is d. *(Stobo, 23/e, pp 790–791.)* Patients with metastatic prostatic carcinoma are treated with endocrine therapy to shrink primary and secondary lesions by depriving prostatic tissue of circulating androgens. Estrogens are no longer recommended because of their negative effects on cardiovascular disease. Most patients now receive a combination of luteinizing hormone–releasing hormone (LHRH) and an antiandrogen (flutamide), which may synergistically block the effect of circulating androgens. Radiotherapy is used for localized disease, but is less effective than prostatectomy. No effective chemotherapy is currently available.

343. The answer is c. *(Fauci, 14/e, pp 731, 744.)* Heparin is a common cause of thrombocytopenia in hospitalized patients. Most cases are due to drug antibody binding to platelets. With a normal spleen on physical exam and normal hemoglobin and white blood cell count, heparin-induced thrombocytopenia would be the likely diagnosis.

344. The answer is c. *(Fauci, 14/e, pp 731, 744.)* Heparin-induced thrombocytopenia is sometimes associated with paradoxical thrombosis called *white clot syndrome.* This syndrome can be fatal unless recognized promptly. Prompt cessation of heparin will reverse thrombocytopenia and heparin-induced thrombosis.

345. The answer is c. *(Fauci, 14/e, pp 419, 868.)* Rifampin causes a reduced-potency effect on Coumadin, requiring higher doses to achieve adequate anticoagulation. When rifampin is stopped, the dose of Coumadin must be reduced or the resulting prothrombin time is likely to be too high. Rifampin and barbiturates accelerate Coumadin clearance by induction of hepatic metabolizing enzymes. Drugs such as disulfiram, metronidazole, and trimethoprim-sulfamethoxazole reduce Coumadin clearance and lead to enhanced potency.

346. The answer is b. *(Fauci, 14/e, pp 2150–2151.)* Patients with hemochromatosis and cirrhosis have a very high incidence of hepatocellular carcinoma. The incidence of this complication is 30% and increases with age. Weight loss and abdominal pain suggest hepatoma in this patient. A CT scan or ultrasound would be indicated. The picture of right upper quadrant pain and elevated alkaline phosphatase would not suggest acute hepatitis or worsening of the cirrhosis caused by hemochromatosis. Primary biliary cirrhosis can cause an obstructive biliary disease, but would be much less likely in this patient.

347. The answer is c. *(Goroll, 3/e, p 983.)* The lesion described is characteristic of leukoplakia. This is a precancerous lesion that requires biopsy. Histologically, these lesions show hyperkeratosis, acanthosis, and atypia. There are homogeneous and nonhomogeneous types. The homogeneous are much more likely to undergo malignant transformation. Oropharyngeal candida would be unlikely to occur in this patient and would appear as a more diffuse, lacy lesion of the buccal mucosa and oropharynx.

348–352. The answers are 348-c, 349-a, 350-b, 351-d, 352-e. *(Fauci, 14/e, p 527.)* Cisplatin produces nephrotoxicity, causing toxic effects to both proximal and distal tubular epithelial cells. Bleomycin can produce diffuse interstitial infiltrates that lead to irreversible pulmonary fibrosis, especially with high cumulative doses and concomitant radiation to lung. Doxorubicin causes cardiac toxicity and congestive heart failure, also dose-related. Left ventricular ejection fraction should be monitored in patients receiving doxorubicin therapy. Vincristine causes neurotoxicity, including foot or wrist drop, cranial nerve palsies, and loss of deep tendon reflexes. Tamoxifen has caused endometrial changes, including hyperplasia, polyps, and endometrial cancer. Any patient who develops vaginal bleeding must be evaluated.

353. The answer is c. *(Fauci, 14/e, pp 648–649.)* Splenomegaly is not typical of sickle cell anemia. Recurrent splenic infarcts may occur, but would result in a small, infarcted spleen. The state of hemolysis resulted in an unconjugated hyperbilirubinemia and low-grade icterus. Anemia and hypoxemia result in a hyperdynamic circulation and a systolic ejection murmur. Ankle ulcers and other chronic skin ulcers may be persistent problems, particularly in those with severe anemia.

354. The answer is e. *(Fauci, 14/e, p 664.)* This 30-year-old black male has developed a hemolytic anemia secondary to an antimalarial drug. Toxins or drugs such as primaquine, sulfamethoxazole, and nitrofurantoin cause hemolysis in patients with G6PD deficiency. It occurs most commonly in blacks. The process is usually self-limited, and no specific treatment other than stopping the drug is necessary. The diagnosis of G6PD deficiency should be considered in any individual, but particularly a male of Mediterranean or African descent who develops an acute hemolytic anemia.

355. The answer is d. *(Fauci, 14/e, p 653–659.)* With anemia and hypersegmented polyps, this patient has a megaloblastic anemia. The evidence for neuropathy makes B_{12} deficiency the diagnosis, since folate deficiency does not cause neuropathy. Pernicious anemia with low B_{12} levels and decreased secretion of intrinsic factor is the most likely cause, although B_{12} deficiency from intestinal malabsorption cannot be ruled out. Antiparietal antibody occurs in 90% of patients with pernicious anemia.

356. The answer is a. *(Fauci, 14/e, p 656.)* The patient has signs and symptoms of adrenal insufficiency, including postural hypotension, hyperpigmentation, hyponatremia, and hyperkalemia. The incidence of pernicious anemia is increased in patients with other autoimmune diseases, such as idiopathic adrenal insufficiency. Vitiligo is also common in these patients. Hyperpigmentation suggests that adrenal insufficiency is not pituitary in origin. In the setting of volume depletion, inappropriate ADH would not be an adequate explanation for the patient's hyponatremia.

357. The answer is b. *(Fauci, 14/e, pp 739–740.)* This patient with gram-negative bacteremia has developed disseminated intravascular coagulation, as evidenced by multiple-site bleeding, thrombocytopenia, fragmented red blood cells on peripheral smear, prolonged PT and PTT, and reduced fibrinogen levels from depletion of coagulation proteins. Initial treatment is directed at correcting the underlying disorder, in this case infection. The use of heparin is somewhat controversial, but generally recommended only in association with acute promyelocytic leukemia.

358. The answer is c. *(Fauci, 14/e, pp 672–675.)* Propylthiouracil can cause a mild or severe leukopenia. When the leukocyte count is less than 1500 cells/mm³ the drug should be discontinued. In the patient described, a white blood cell count must be determined in order to further manage the patient. Blood cultures may also be in order, but this is not the most important initial step.

359–361. The answers are 358-a, 359-c, 360-d. *(Fauci, 14/e, pp 638–645, 1518.)* The alcoholic patient being treated for tuberculosis has sideroblastic anemia. Both ethanol and isoniazid inhibit one or more steps in heme synthesis. The disorder results in ringed sideroblasts, nucleated erythroid precursors, a hypochromic, microcytic anemia, and the characteristic increase in serum iron and transferrin saturation.

Low serum iron and elevated iron-binding capacity would be present in anemia of iron deficiency. All of the anemias listed are microcytic, hypochromic, with the exception of anemia of renal disease. The anemia of renal disease is a normocytic, normochromic anemia. The diseased kidney is unable to secrete adequate amounts of erythropoietin.

362–365. The answers are 362-b, 363-e, 364-f, 365-c. *(Fauci, 14/e, pp 684–695.)* The sticklike primary granules described are called *Auer bodies.* They are seen in 10 to 20% of patients with AML and are diagnostic. Acute promyelocytic leukemia and subtype of AML (M3) is the leukemia associated with DIC. DIC is usually present at the time of diagnosis and may worsen during chemotherapy. Cytoplasmic projections seen on leukemic cells in peripheral smear and bone marrow occur in hairy cell leukemia. Cells have an eccentrically placed nucleus with foamy cytoplasm.

In 90% of patients with ALL, leukemic lymphoblasts contain a nuclear enzyme terminal called *deoxynucleotidyl transferase* (tdt). This transferase occurs in about 20% of patients with AML.

NEUROLOGY

DIRECTIONS: Each item below contains a question or incomplete statement followed by suggested responses. Select the **one best** response to each question.

366. A 30-year-old male complains of unilateral headaches. He complains of rhinorrhea and tearing of the eye on the side of the headache. Episodes are precipitated by alcohol. Headaches may become a problem for weeks to months, after which a headache-free period occurs. The most likely diagnosis is

a. Migraine
b. Cluster
c. Sinusitis
d. Tension headache

367. A 35-year-old previously healthy woman complains of a severe, excruciating headache and then has a transient loss of consciousness. There are no focal neurologic findings. The next step in evaluation would be

a. CT scan without contrast
b. CT scan with contrast
c. Carotid angiogram
d. Holter monitor

368. A 70-year-old male complains of the sudden onset of syncope. It occurs without warning and with no sweating, dizziness, or light-headedness. He believes episodes tend to occur when turning his head too quickly or sometimes when shaving. The best way to make a definitive diagnosis in this patient would be

a. ECG
b. Carotid massage with ECG monitoring
c. Holter monitor
d. Electrophysiologic studies to evaluate the AV node

Items 369–371

369. A 30-year-old male complains of leg weakness and parasthesias of the arm and leg. Five years previously he had a episode of transient visual loss. On physical exam, there is hyperreflexia, bilateral Babinski signs, and cerebellar dysmetria with poor finger-to-nose movement. When asked to look to the right, the left eye does not move normally past the midline. There is nystagmus noted in the abducting eye. A more detailed history suggests the patient has had episodes of gait difficulty that have resolved spontaneously. He has no systemic symptoms of fever or weight loss. The most likely diagnosis in this patient is

a. Multiple sclerosis
b. Vitamin B_{12} deficiency
c. Systemic lupus erythematosis
d. Hypochondriasis

370. The best test to pursue this diagnosis is

a. Lumbar puncture
b. MRI
c. Quantitative IgG levels
d. CSF myelin protein

371. Which of the following best summarizes the role of interferon beta for this disease?

a. It can reduce the number of relapses and the appearance of new lesions on MRI
b. It can cure one-third of patients
c. It improves survival
d. It improves patients symptoms and has no significant side effects

Items 372–373

372. A 50-year-old male has complained of slowly progressive weakness over several months. Walking has become more difficult, as has using his hands. There are no sensory, bowel, or bladder complaints. There are no problems in thinking, speech, or vision. Examination shows distal muscle weakness with muscle wasting and fasciculations. There are also upper motor neuron signs, including extensor plantar reflexes and hyperreflexia in wasted-muscle groups. The most likely diagnosis is

a. Polymyositis
b. Duchenne muscular dystrophy
c. Amyotrophic lateral sclerosis
d. Myasthenia gravis

373. The laboratory test most likely to be abnormal in this patient is

a. Cerebrospinal fluid white blood cell count
b. Sensory conduction studies
c. CT scan brain
d. Electromyography

374. A 20-year-old woman complains of weakness that is worse in the afternoon, worse during repetitive activity, and improved by rest. When fatigued, the patient is unable to "hold her head up," speak, or chew her food. On physical exam, there is no loss of reflexes, sensation, or coordination. The underlying pathogenesis of this disease is

a. Serum antiacetylcholine receptor antibodies causing neuromuscular transmission failure
b. Destruction of anterior horn cells by virus
c. Progressive muscular atrophy
d. Demyelinating disease

375. The diagnosis of myasthenia gravis is made by a positive edrophonium test, repetitive nerve-stimulation test of a weak muscle, and antiacetylcholine receptor antibody assay. MRI of the mediastinum is now indicated to

a. Rule out tuberculosis before starting prednisone
b. Rule out thymoma
c. Look for small cell carcinoma and Lambert-Eaton syndrome
d. Rule out sarcoidosis

DIRECTIONS: Each group of questions below consists of lettered headings followed by a set of numbered items. For each numbered item select the **one** lettered heading with which it is most closely associated. Each lettered heading may be used once, more than once, or not at all.

Items 376–378

Match the clinical description with the most likely disease process.

a. Parkinson's disease
b. Wilson's disease
c. Huntington's chorea
d. Dystonia
e. Essential tremor
f. Tic

376. An 18-year-old male with resting tremor, bradykinesia, rigidity, drooling; deposits in cornea; abnormal liver function tests.

377. An elderly patient with bradykinesia, micrographia, and resting tremor.

378. Rapid, writhing movements in a 40-year-old associated with dementia.

DIRECTIONS: Each item below contains a question or incomplete statement followed by suggested responses. Select the **one best** response to each question.

Items 379–380

379. Three weeks after an upper respiratory illness, a 25-year-old male develops weakness of his arms and legs over several days. On physical exam he is tachypneic, with shallow respirations and symmetric muscle weakness in both arms and legs. There is no obvious sensory deficit, but motor reflexes cannot be elicited. The most likely diagnosis is

a. Myasthenia graves
b. Multiple sclerosis
c. Guillain-Barré syndrome
d. Dermatomyositis
e. Diabetes mellitus

380. The workup of this patient is most likely to show

a. Acellular spinal fluid with high protein
b. Abnormal EMG that shows axonal degeneration
c. Positive Tensilon test
d. Elevated CPK
e. Respiratory alkalosis by arterial blood gases

Items 381–384

Match the clinical description with the most likely disease process.

a. Senile dementia of the Alzheimer's type
b. Multi-infarct dementia
c. Vitamin B_{12} deficiency
d. Delirium
e. Creutzfeldt-Jakob disease
f. Normal pressure hydrocephalus

381. An 80-year-old develops steady, progressive memory and cognitive deficit over two years. He has normal blood pressure, no focal neurologic findings, and workup for dementia is negative.

382. A 60-year-old woman admitted for urinary retention develops acute confusion and disorientation.

383. A 70-year-old male with history of hypertension and previous history of stroke; presents with new focal findings and acute worsening of cognitive function.

384. A 50-year-old presents with rapidly progressive change in mental status over three months; has episodes of myoclonus and abnormal EEG.

Items 385–387

	WBC	% Polys	Glucose (mg/dL)	Protein (mg/dL)	Pressure
a.	10,000	99%	20	60	30
b.	200	0%	20	55	30
c.	200	0%	80	30	8
d.	0	0%	80	100	40
e.	3	0%	80	20	8

385. Fever, stiff neck; CSF has positive quellung reaction

386. Patient on high dose corticosteroids; positive india ink stain

387. History of dental abscess; has focal neurologic findings and low-grade fever

Items 388–390

Match each symptom or sign with the appropriate diagnosis.

a. Tension headache
b. Cluster headache
c. Migraine headache
d. Temporal arteritis
e. Brain tumor
f. Sinusitis
g. Temporomandibular joint dysfunction
h. Tic douloureux

388. Bilateral, bandlike sensation around head; dull, steady pain may last days, weeks; may have occipital or nuchal soreness

389. Unilateral, nonthrobbing headache; more common in men; nasal stuffiness and lacrimation

390. Unilateral headache with localized scalp tenderness in older patient; may have transient visual loss

DIRECTIONS: Each question below contains five suggested responses. Select the **one best** response to each question.

391. A 45-year-old woman presents to her physician with an eight-month history of gradually increasing limb weakness. She first noticed difficulty climbing stairs, then problems rising from chairs, walking more than half a block, and, finally, lifting her arms above shoulder level. Aside from some difficulty swallowing, she has no ocular, bulbar, or sphincter problems and no sensory complaints. Family history is negative for neurological disease. Examination reveals significant proximal limb and neck muscle weakness with minimal atrophy, normal sensory findings, and intact deep tendon reflexes. The most likely diagnosis in this patient is

a. Polymyositis
b. Cervical myelopathy
c. Myasthenia gravis
d. Mononeuropathy multiplex
e. Limb-girdle muscular dystrophy

392. A 55-year-old diabetic woman suddenly develops weakness of the left side of her face as well as of her right arm and leg. She also has diplopia on left lateral gaze. The responsible lesion is probably located in the

a. Right cerebral hemisphere
b. Left cerebral hemisphere
c. Right side of the brainstem
d. Left side of the brainstem
e. Right medial longitudinal fasciculus

393. Which of the following is *not* a recognized neurological complication of HIV infection?

a. Dementia
b. Cerebral toxoplasmosis
c. CNS astrocytoma
d. Myelopathy
e. Chronic inflammatory polyneuropathy

394. Which of the following symptoms would suggest that the headaches suffered by a patient were due to migraine?

a. Numbness or tingling of the left face, lips, and hand lasting for 5 to 15 minutes, followed by a throbbing headache
b. An increasingly throbbing headache associated with unilateral visual loss and generalized muscle aches
c. A continuous headache associated with sleepiness, nausea, ataxia, and incoordination of the right upper limb
d. An intense, left retroorbital headache associated with transient left-sided ptosis and rhinorrhea
e. A visual field defect that persists following cessation of a unilateral headache

395. Diffuse hyperreflexia in a limb that is markedly atrophic and weak can be seen in which of the following disorders?

a. Brachial plexus neuropathy involving the upper trunk
b. Recent cerebral infarction with hemiparesis
c. Cervical radiculopathy
d. Multiple sclerosis
e. Amyotrophic lateral sclerosis

396. Which of the following statements about the treatment of Parkinson's disease is correct?

a. Limb and facial dyskinesias are unusual side effects of chronic levodopa therapy
b. Levodopa treatment, while ameliorating symptoms, does not alter the natural history of the disease
c. Bromocriptine works by increasing the release of dopamine from the substantia nigra
d. Use of trihexyphenidyl and benztropine mesylate have minimal side effects in the elderly

DIRECTIONS: Each group of questions below consists of lettered headings followed by a set of numbered items. For each numbered item select the **one** lettered heading with which it is most closely associated. Each lettered heading may be used once, more than once, or not at all.

Items 397–400

Match each description below with the appropriate dementia-causing disorder.

a. Hypothyroid dementia
b. Normal pressure hydrocephalus
c. Multi-infarct dementia
d. Creutzfeldt-Jakob disease
e. Alzheimer's disease

397. Aphasia, agnosia, and apraxia are common; memory loss prominent; familial occurrence well documented; silver-staining neuritic plaques seen throughout cortex

398. Stuttering course; often associated with distinct focal neurological events; pseudobulbar palsy common; hypertension often present

399. Rapid progression; myoclonic jerks; distinctive EEG pattern; occurrence in those receiving injections of human growth hormone

400. Unsteadiness of gait with impairment of balance; urinary incontinence; may follow subarachnoid hemorrhage; CT scan important for diagnosis

Items 401–404

a. Absence (petit mal) seizures
b. Complex partial seizures
c. Simple partial
d. Atonic
e. Myoclonic seizure

401. Postictal confusion

402. Three-per-second spike-and-wave discharges

403. Déjà vu experiences

404. Loss of postural muscle tone and brief loss of consciousness

Items 405–408

a. Guillain-Barré syndrome
b. Myasthenia gravis
c. Amyotrophic lateral sclerosis
d. Duchenne muscular dystrophy

405. Limb weakness, elevated CSF protein, normal CSF white cell count

406. Response to edrophonium, reflexes normal

407. Asymmetric muscle weakness, stiffness; hyperreflexia

408. Pseudohypertrophy, Gowers' manuever

NEUROLOGY

Answers

366. The answer is b. *(Stobo, 23d edition, pp 841–843.)* This headache is most consistent with a type of neurovascular headache called *cluster headache.* These occur in young men, have a characteristic periodicity, or cluster, and cause lacrimation, nasal stuffiness, and sometimes conjunctival inflammation. Migraines tend not to come and go in this manner. They are more throbbing and more likely to be associated with nausea and vomiting. Sinusitis is usually bilateral with associated fever, purulent discharge. Tension headaches are usually described as bandlike, without lacrimation or nasal congestion.

367. The answer is a. *(Stobo, 23/e, pp 849–850.)* An excruciating headache with syncope requires evaluation for subarachnoid hemorrhage. About 80% of patients will have enough blood to be visualized on an non-contrast CT scan. If the scan is normal a lumbar puncture would be the next step to establish the presence of subarachnoid blood. A contrast CT scan sometimes obscures the diagnosis because in an enhanced scan, normal arteries may be mistaken for clotted blood.

368. The answer is b. *(Stobo, 23/e, pp 73–74.)* When syncope occurs in an older patient as a result of head turning, wearing a tight shirt collar, or shaving over the neck area, carotid sinus hypersensitivity should be considered. Some consider the process to be quite rare. Gentle massage of one carotid sinus at a time may show a period of asystole. This should be performed in a controlled setting, as it is not without risks.

369. The answer is a. *(Stobo, 23/e, pp 857–870.)* This young man has had an episode of transient blindness, likely due to optic neuritis. This transient loss of vision in one eye occurs in about 25 to 40% of multiple sclerosis patients. (A similar presentation can occur in SLE, sarcoidosis, and syphilis.) In addition, the patient gives a history of a relapsing-remitting process. There are abnormal signs of peripheral nerve, cerebellar, and upper motor neuron disease. Signs and symptoms therefore suggest multiple lesions. This would make multiple sclerosis the most likely diagnosis. There are no systemic symptoms to suggest SLE. B_{12} deficiency could explain all the neurologic deficits noted. Objective physical exam data rules out hypochondriasis—a diagnosis sometimes inappropriately given to the MS patient.

370. The answer is b. *(Stobo, 23/e, pp 857–870.)* All patients with suspected multiple sclerosis should have an MRI of the brain. MRI is sensitive in defining demyelinating lesions in the brain and spinal cord. Most patients do not need lumbar puncture or spinal fluid analysis for diagnosis, although 70% have elevated IgG levels, and myelin basic protein does appear in the CSF during exacerbations.

371. The answer is a. *(Stobo, 23/e, pp 862–863.)* Interferon beta reduces the number of exacerbations of MS and decreases new lesions seen on MRI. It does not cure the disease. Interferon beta can cause side effects, particularly a flulike syndrome.

372. The answer is c. *(Stobo, 23/e, pp 894–895.)* The disease described involves motor neurons exclusively. Amyotrophic lateral sclerosis affects both upper and motor neurons. In this patient, there is upper and lower motor neuron involvement without sensory deficit. Peripheral neuropathy and dementia do not occur. Duchenne muscular dystrophy occurs at a younger age and involves proximal muscle weakness and not motor neurons. Polymyositis is also primarily a muscle disease. Myasthenia gravis would not cause hyperreflexia or Babinski reflex. It is a disease of muscle weakness characterized by fatigability.

373. The answer is d. *(Stobo, 23/e, p 895.)* EMG would show widespread denervation potentials. The other tests would be normal.

374. The answer is a. *(Stobo, 23/e, pp 896–897.)* Myasthenia gravis results from a reduction in the number of junctional acetylcholine receptors as a result of autoantibodies. Antibodies cross-link these receptors, causing a facilitation of endocytosis and degradation in lysosomes.

375. The answer is b. *(Stobo, 23/e, pp 896–897.)* Ten percent of myasthenia patients have thymic tumors. Surgical removal of all thymomas is necessary because of local tumor spread. Sarcoidosis causes peripheral neuropathy, aseptic meningitis, but not a myasthenia syndrome. Small cell carcinoma is associated with Lambert-Eaton syndrome, a paraneoplastic syndrome similar to myasthenia. A chest x-ray would be sufficient to screen for malignancy or infection.

376–378. The answers are 376-b, 377-a, 378-c. *(Stobo, 5/e, pp 853–856.)* A movement disorder in itself in a young person suggests Wilson's disease. This is an autosomal recessive disorder in which a deficiency in the copper-binding protein, ceruloplasmin, results in copper deposition in tissue. Copper deposition in the basal ganglia causes tremor and rigidity. Copper deposition in the eye produces the Kayser-Fleischer ring. Deposition in the liver causes cirrhosis and hepatitis. The diagnosis of Parkinson's is based on resting tremor, cogwheel rigidity, and bradykinesia. Micrographia, small handwriting, is also characteristic. Huntington's chorea is suspected in association with dementia and rapid, nonrhythmic movements. The disease is autosomal dominant and presents in the third or fourth decade of life. There are often slow, writhing movements called *athetosis*.

379. The answer is c. *(Fauci, 14/e, pp 2462–2463.)* This young man presents with an acute symmetrical polyneuropathy characteristic of the patient with Guillain-Barré syndrome. This is a demyelinating polyneuropathy that is often preceded by a viral illness. Characteristically, there is little sensory involvement, and about 30% of patients require ventilatory assistance.

Dermatomyositis usually presents insidiously with proximal muscle weakness. Myasthenia gravis also presents insidiously with muscle weakness worsened by repetitive use. Diplopia, ptosis, and facial weakness are common first complaints. Multiple sclerosis causes demyelinating lesions disseminated in time and space—and would not occur in this acute, symmetrical manner.

Diabetes mellitus can cause a variety of neuropathies, but would not be rapidly progressive as in this patient.

380. The answer is a. *(Fauci, 14/e, p 2462.)* Guillain-Barré syndrome is characterized by an elevated CSF protein with few if any white blood cells. EMG would show a demyelinating process with nonuniform slowing and conduction block. Arterial blood gases would show a respiratory acidosis secondary to hypoventilation. CPK levels should be normal, as there is little involvement of muscle in this disease process.

381–384. The answers are 381-a, 382-d, 383-b, 384-e. *(Fauci, 14/e, pp 2348–2355.)* The 80-year-old patient with progressive, steady memory loss and cognitive dysfunction over two years has not been found to have a reversible cause of dementia by standard workup. The great majority of such patients have senile dementia of the Alzheimer type. At present, there is no definitive method of premortem diagnosis, but characteristic histologic findings of neurofibrillary tangles and neuritic plaques would be noted at autopsy. The 60-year-old woman has developed an acute clouding of consciousness and an acute confusional state described as *delirium.* This may occur in association with infection, drug effect, acute illness, or change in environment.

The 70-year-old with hypertension and previous stroke is most likely to have a multi-infarct dementia. This is a progressive stepwise deterioration, usually the result of recurrent bilateral cerebral emboli. Focal findings are common, including hemiparesis, extensor plantar responses, and pseudobulbar palsy. The patient with rapidly progressive dementia and myoclonus must be evaluated for Creutzfeldt-Jakob disease. This is a transmissible neurodegenerative dementia that shows a typical EEG pattern of periodic bilaterally synchronous sharp-wave complexes.

385–387. The answers are 385-a, 386-b, 387-d. *(Gantz, 4/e pp 151–157.)* The fever and stiff neck with a positive quellung reaction on CSF proves the diagnosis of pneumococcal meningitis. The CSF of a patient with bacterial meningitis will show thousands of white blood cells, with more than 90% being polymorphonuclear leukocytes. The protein is always elevated, and glucose is usually lower than normal. The patient on high-dose corticosteroids and a CSF with a positive india ink stain has cryptococcal meningitis. Cryptococcal meningitis patients usually have a lymphocytic meningitis also, with an elevated CSF protein and low CSF sugar.

The patient with focal findings and a history of dental abscess has a brain abscess. Lumbar puncture is contraindicated in the disease, but would usually show only a small number of white blood cells, if any, and a high protein and elevated CSF pressure.

388–390. The answers are 388-a, 389-b, 390-d. *(Fauci, 14/e, pp 68–72, 2307–2310.)* Tension headaches are the leading cause of chronic headaches, and 90% are bilateral. Headaches are described as dull, constricting, bandlike. Associated tenderness may be present.

Cluster headaches such as migraine and temporal arteritis are unilateral headaches. Cluster headaches differ from migraines in that they are nonthrobbing and are more common in men.

Temporal arteritis may cause scalp tenderness localized to the involved vessel. It is primarily a disease of the elderly. Blindness caused by occlusion of the ophthalmic artery is the feared complication.

391. The answer is a. *(Fauci, 14/e, pp 1896–1897.)* Polymyositis is an acquired myopathy characterized by subacute symmetrical weakness of proximal limb and trunk muscles that progresses over several weeks or months. When a characteristic skin rash occurs, the disease is known as *dermatomyositis.* In addition to progressive proximal limb weakness, the patient often presents with dysphagia and neck muscle weakness. Up to one-half of cases with polymyositis-dermatomyositis may have, in addition, features of connective tissue diseases (rheumatoid arthritis, lupus erythematosus, scleroderma, Sjögren's syndrome). Laboratory findings include an elevated serum CK level, an EMG showing myopathic potentials with fibrillations, and a muscle biopsy showing necrotic muscle fibers and inflammatory infiltrates. Polymyositis is clinically distinguished from the muscular dystrophies by its less prolonged course and lack of family history. It is distinguished from myasthenia gravis by its lack of ocular muscle involvement, absence of variability in strength over hours or days, and lack of response to cholinesterase inhibitor drugs.

392. The answer is d. *(Fauci, 14/e, pp 2327–2339.)* This patient has weakness of the left face and the contralateral (right) arm and leg, commonly called a *crossed hemiplegia.* Such crossed syndromes are characteristic of brainstem lesions. In this case, the lesion is an infarct localized to the left inferior pons and caused by occlusion of a branch of the basilar artery. The infarct has damaged the left sixth and seventh cranial nerves or nuclei in the left pons with resultant diplopia on left lateral gaze and left facial weakness. Also damaged in the left pons is the left corticospinal tract, proximal to its decussation in the medulla; this damage causes weakness in the right arm and leg. This classic presentation is called the *Millard-Gubler syndrome.*

393. The answer is c. *(Fauci, 14/e, pp 1820–1830.)* Neurological complications of AIDS are either due to primary infection with the AIDS virus (HIV) or secondary to immunosuppression and occur in at least one-third of patients with AIDS. A common occurrence in later stages is the AIDS dementia complex, a progressive dementia associated with motor abnormalities that is felt to be due to direct infection with HIV. Other CNS complications related to immunosuppression include cerebral toxoplasmosis, primary CNS lymphoma, herpes zoster encephalitis, and infections due to tuberculosis, syphilis, cytomegalovirus (CMV), and cryptococcus. A myelopathy with vacuolar degeneration is common, and a variety of neuropathic conditions have been described, including a distal sensory polyneuropathy and both the acute (Guillain-Barré syndrome) and chronic forms of inflammatory demyelinating polyneuropathy.

394. The answer is a. *(Fauci, 14/e, pp 2307–2310.)* The differential diagnosis of headaches associated with neurological or visual dysfunction is important because it encompasses a variety of disorders, some quite serious and other relatively benign. Classic (or neurological) migraine is generally a familial disorder that begins in childhood or early adult life. Typically, the onset of an episode is marked by the progression of a neurological disturbance over 5 to 15 minutes, followed by a unilateral (or occasionally bilateral) throbbing headache for from several hours up to a day. The most common neurological disturbance involves formed or unformed flashes of light that impair vision in one of the visual fields (*scintillating scotoma*). Other possible neurological symptoms include numbness and tingling of the unilateral face, lips, and hand; weakness of an arm or leg; mild aphasia; and mental confusion. The transience of the neurological symptoms distinguishes migraine from other, more serious conditions that cause headaches. Persistence of a visual field defect, speech disturbance, or mild hemiparesis suggests a focal lesion (e.g., arteriovenous malformation with hemorrhage or infarct). In the case of persistent ataxia, limb incoordination, and nausea, one should consider a posterior fossa (possibly cerebellar) mass lesion. Monocular visual loss in an elderly patient with throbbing headaches should initiate a search for cranial (temporal) arteritis. This should include a sedimentation rate (usually elevated) and a temporal artery biopsy (which would show a giant cell arteritis). Fifty percent of these patients have the generalized muscle aches seen with polymyalgia rheumatica. Unilateral orbital or retroorbital headaches that occur nightly for a period of two to eight weeks are characteristic of cluster headaches. These headaches are often associated with ipsilateral injection of the conjunctivum, nasal stuffiness, rhinorrhea, and, less commonly, miosis, ptosis, and cheek edema. Although both migraine and cluster headaches may respond to treatment with ergotamine, they are generally considered to be distinct entities.

395. The answer is e. *(Fauci, 14/e, pp 2368–2370.)* Diffuse hyperreflexia of an arm or leg indicates upper motor neuron dysfunction at a segmental level above that which supplies the involved limbs. Although weakness can be present with both upper and lower motor neuron lesions, marked muscle atrophy indicates axonal dysfunction in the lower motor neurons that innervate the limb's muscles. Thus, the combination of limb hyperreflexia and significant muscle atrophy can be seen only in conditions that cause both upper and lower motor neuron dysfunction of multiple segments. Amyotrophic lateral sclerosis is such a condition. Both brachial plexus neuropathy and cervical radiculopathy affect only the lower motor neurons and cause segmental weakness, atrophy, and depressed or absent tendon reflexes. Cerebral infarction and multiple sclerosis usually disrupt the corticospinal tracts unilaterally or bilaterally; they cause weakness and spastic hyperreflexia with little or no atrophy.

396. The answer is b. *(Fauci, 14/e, pp 2356–2359.)* Parkinson's disease (PD) is marked by depletion of dopamine-rich cells in the substantia nigra. The resulting decrease in striatal dopamine is the basis for the classic symptoms of rigidity, bradykinesia, and tremor. By far the most widely used treatment for PD has been the drug levodopa. Levodopa is converted to dopamine in the substantia nigra and then transported to the striatum, where it stimulates dopamine receptors. This is the basis for the drug's clinical effect on PD. Levodopa is usually administered with carbidopa (a decarboxylase inhibitor) in one pill (Sinemet), which prevents levodopa's destruction in the blood and allows it to be given at a dose that is lower and less likely to cause nausea and vomiting. The major problems with levodopa have been (1) significant limb and facial dyskinesias in most patients on chronic therapy and (2) the fact that levodopa treats PD only symptomatically, and the disease process of neuronal loss in the substantia nigra continues despite drug treatment.

Other drugs can be used in the treatment of PD. Anticholinergic agents, such as trihexyphenidyl (Artane) and benztropine mesylate

(Cogentin), work by restoring the balance between striatal dopamine and acetylcholine. They can have significant anticholinergic effects on the CNS, including confusional states and hallucinations. Bromocriptine and pergolide are dopamine agonists that work directly by stimulating dopamine receptors in the striatum; side effects of these drugs are similar to those of levodopa. Selegiline (Eldepryl) is a selective monoamine oxidase-B (MAO-B) inhibitor that blocks the breakdown of intracerebral dopamine.

397–400. The answers are 397-e, 398-c, 399-d, 400-b. *(Fauci, 14/e, pp 144–148, 2348–2351, 2352–2353.)* Alzheimer's disease, which is the most common degenerative disease of the brain, usually occurs in patients in their late fifties and older. The disease is highlighted by progressive dementia, which begins with memory deficits and personality changes and progresses to involve disorders of cerebral function, including aphasias, agnosias, and apraxias. Pathological changes in the cerebral cortex include neuritic (senile) plaques, neurofibrillary tangles within nerve cells, and granulovacuolar degeneration of neurons. Multi-infarct, or arteriosclerotic, dementia indicates intellectual impairment as a result of multiple cerebral strokes. Patients usually have a stuttering course with a temporal profile of distinct neurological events (indicating strokes) associated with progression of dementia. Multiple infarcts may also produce a picture of pseudobulbar palsy (i.e., slurred speech, dysphagia, and emotional overflow).

Creutzfeldt-Jakob disease, also known as *subacute spongiform encephalopathy,* is a nervous system disease marked by a rapidly progressive dementia, diffuse myoclonic jerks, and cerebellar ataxia. Many patients have a distinctive EEG pattern of generalized sharp-wave complexes that recur at a rate of one per second. Gibbs has shown that the disease can be transmitted to primates by injecting them with diseased brain tissue. Latrogenic disease has also occurred in patients who received growth hormone prepared from pooled cadaveric pituitary glands.

Normal pressure hydrocephalus (NPH) is thought to be due to nonprogressive meningeal and ependymal diseases and is characterized by enlarged ventricles with minimal or no brain atrophy. Patients with NPH manifest a clinical triad of progressive gait disorder, urinary incontinence, and dementia. CT scanning or radionuclide cisternography can usually verify the diagnosis of NPH, which may be cured by a ventricular shunt procedure.

401–404. The answers are 401-b, 402-a, 403-b, 404-d. *(Fauci, 4/e, pp 2312–2316.)* Typical absence, or petit mal, seizure is the most characteristic epilepsy of childhood, with onset usually between age 4 and the early teens. Attacks, which may occur as frequently as several hundred in a day, consist of sudden interruptions of consciousness. The child stares, stops talking or responding, often displays eye fluttering, and commonly shows automatisms such as lip smacking and fumbling movements of the fingers. Attacks end in 2 to 10 seconds with the patient fully alert and able to resume activities. The characteristic EEG abnormality associated with attacks is three-per-second spike-and-wave activity.

Complex partial seizures, also known as *psychomotor seizures*, are characterized by complex auras with psychic experiences and periods of impaired consciousness with altered motor behavior. Common psychic experiences include illusions, visual or auditory hallucinations, feelings of familiarity (déjà vu) or strangeness (*jamais vu*), and fear or anxiety. Motor components include automatisms (e.g., lip smacking) and so-called automatic behavior (walking around in a daze, undressing in public). The brain lesion is usually in the temporal lobe, less commonly in the frontal lobe, and is often manifest as a focal epileptiform abnormality on EEG. Postictal confusion or drowsiness is the rule. Simple partial seizures cause focal motor, sensory, or psychic symptoms without loss of consciousness. Atonic seizures are marked by loss of postural tone. Brief loss of consciousness can occur but there is no postictal confusion.

405–408. The answers are 405-c, 406-b, 407-c, 408-d. *(Fauci, 14/e, pp 2462, 2368–2370, 2469–2470, 2473.)* Guillain-Barré syndrome, also known as *acute inflammatory polyradiculoneuropathy*, is an acute demyelinating polyneuropathy characterized by diffuse limb weakness that progresses to a maximum deficit over two to three weeks. As the syndrome develops, typical findings include proximal and distal limb weakness, ophthalmoplegias with facial weakness, areflexia, and, frequently, respiratory insufficiency. The CSF shows an elevated protein with normal white cell count (albuminocytologic dissociation), and the EMG/nerve conduction study indicates a demyelinating neuropathy.

Myasthenia gravis is a disease of the neuromuscular junction that results in fluctuating and sometimes persistent weakness of ocular, bulbar, limb, and respiratory muscles. More than 90% of patients develop extraocular palsies or ptosis, and 80% develop some weakness of the muscles of facial expression, mastication, swallowing, or speech. Diaphragmatic muscle weakness can lead to respiratory insufficiency. Sensory function and deep tendon reflexes are preserved. Weakened muscles usually improve dramatically upon administration of parenteral anticholinesterase drugs such as edrophonium (Tensilon).

Duchenne muscular dystrophy is present at birth, but does not manifest itself until age 3 to 5. Gowers' manuever describes the child, who after falling, climbs upright by placing hands on lower legs. Calf muscles become replaced by fat and connective tissue, giving the appearance of hypertrophy.

In amyotrophic lateral sclerosis, weakness is characteristically asymmetrical due to lower motor neuron denervation. Patients with reflex hyperactivity secondary to corticospinal involvement complain of muscle stiffness out of proportion to weakness.

DERMATOLOGY

DIRECTIONS: Each item below contains a question or incomplete statement followed by suggested responses. Select the **one best** response to each question.

409. A 20-year-old woman complains of skin problems and is noted to have erythematous papules on her face with blackheads (open comedones) and whiteheads (closed comedones). She has also had cystic lesions. She is prescribed a topical tretinoin (Retin-A), but without a totally acceptable result. Which of the following is correct?

a. Intralesional triamcinolone should be avoided due to its systemic effects
b. Systemically administered isoretinoin therapy could not be considered unless concomitant contraceptive therapy is provided
c. Antimicrobial therapy is of no value since bacteria are not part of the pathogenesis of the process
d. Isoretinoin is without important side effects as long as it is not used in sexually active women

410. A 22-year-old male presents with a six-month history of a red, nonpruritic rash over the trunk, scalp, elbows, and knees. These eruptions are more likely to occur during stressful periods and have occurred at sites of skin injury. On exam, sharply demarcated plaques are seen with a thick scale. Which of the following statements is correct?

a. Lesions are contagious and contact should be carefully avoided
b. The patient is allergic to metals
c. The clinical description is most consistent with psoriasis
d. The rash is unrelated to stress

411. A 25-year-old has complained of fever and myalgias for five days and now has developed a macular rash over his palms and soles with some petechial lesions. The patient has recently returned from a summer camping trip in the Great Smoky Mountains. The most likely cause of the rash is

a. Contact dermatitis
b. Sexual exposure
c. Tick exposure
d. Contaminated stream

412. A 17-year-old female presents with a pruritic rash localized to the wrist. Papules and vesicles are noted in a bandlike pattern, with slight oozing from some lesions. The most likely cause of the rash is

a. Herpes simplex
b. Shingles
c. Contact dermatitis
d. Seborrheic dermatitis

Items 413–414

413. A 35-year-old woman has developed an itchy rash over her back, legs, and trunk several hours after swimming in a lake. Erythematous, edematous papules are noted. The wheals vary in size. There are no mucosal lesions and no swelling of the lips. The most likely diagnosis is

a. Urticaria
b. Folliculitis
c. Erythema multiforme
d. Erythema chronicum migrans

414. The treatment of choice for this patient would be

a. Epinephrine
b. Intravenous glucocorticoids
c. Antihistamines and avoidance of offending agent
d. Aspirin

415. A 30-year-old black female has had a history of cough, and a chest x-ray shows bilateral hilar lymphadenopathy. A biopsy shows noncaseating granuloma. The skin lesion most consistent with the patient's diagnosis would be

a. Seborrheic keratosis
b. Asymmetric pigmented lesion with irregular border
c. Erythema nodosum
d. Umbilicated, dome-shaped yellow papules

Items 416–417

416. An elderly, homeless male is evaluated for anemia. On exam he has purpura and ecchymoses of the legs. Perifollicular papules and perifollicular hemorrhages are also noted. There is swelling and bleeding of gums around the patient's teeth. There is tenderness around a hematoma of the calf. The most likely diagnosis is

a. Elder abuse
b. Scurvy
c. Pellagra
d. Beriberi

417. The best approach to the management of this patient would be

a. Obtain platelet ascorbic acid level and give ascorbic acid while in hospital
b. Discharge with dietary consult
c. Give folic acid
d. Obtain plasma tryptophan

418. This 50-year-old woman has developed pink macules and papules on the hands and forearms in association with a sore throat. The lesions are target-like, with the centers a dusty violet. A diagnosis of erythema multiforme is made. The most important information obtained from this patient's history is

a. The patient has been using tampons
b. The patient is taking Dilantin
c. The patient has never had measles
d. No other family members have a sore throat

419. This 25-year-old female with blonde hair and fair complexion complains of a mole. The lesion is on the upper back. The lesion is 6 mm, darkly pigmented, and asymmetric, with a very irregular border. The next step in management would be

a. Tell patient to avoid sunlight
b. Follow the lesion for any evidence of growth
c. Obtain metastatic workup
d. Obtain full-thickness excisional biopsy
e. Obtain shave biopsy

420. This 39-year-old male with a prior history of myocardial infarction complains of yellow bumps on his elbows and buttocks. Yellow-colored cutaneous plaques are noted in those areas. The next step in evaluation of this patient would be

a. Biopsy of skin lesions
b. Lipid profile
c. Uric acid levels
d. Chest x-ray to evaluate for sarcoidosis

421. A 15-year-old girl complains of a low-grade fever, malaise, conjunctivitis, coryza, and cough. After this prodromal phase, a rash of discrete pink macules begins on her face and extends to her hands and feet. She is also noted to have small red spots on her palate. The cause of her rash is

a. Toxic shock syndrome
b. Gonococcal bacteremia
c. Reiter's syndrome
d. Rubeola (measles)
e. Rubella (German measles)

422. A 17-year-old girl noted a 2-cm, annular, pink, scaly lesion on her thigh. In the next two weeks she developed several smaller, oval, pink lesions with a fine collarette of scale. They seem to run in the body folds and mainly involve the trunk, although a few are on the upper arms and thighs. There is no adenopathy and no oral lesions. The most likely diagnosis is

a. Tinea versicolor
b. Psoriasis
c. Lichen planus
d. Pityriasis rosea
e. Secondary syphilis

423. A 45-year-old man with Parkinson's disease has macular areas of erythema and scaling behind the ears and on the scalp, eyebrows, glabella, nasal labial folds, and central chest. The diagnosis is

a. Tinea versicolor
b. Psoriasis
c. Seborrheic dermatitis
d. Atopic dermatitis
e. Dermatophyte infection

424. A 20-year-old white man has noted an uneven tan on his upper back and chest. On examination he has many circular, lighter macules with a barely visible scale that coalesce into larger areas. The best test procedure to establish the diagnosis is a

a. Punch biopsy
b. Potassium hydroxide (KOH) microscopic examination
c. Dermatophyte test medium (DTM) culture for fungus
d. Serological test for syphilis
e. Tzank smear

425. A 33-year-old fair-skinned woman has telangiectasias of the cheeks and nose along with red papules and occasional pustules. She also appears to have a conjunctivitis because of dilated scleral vessels. She reports frequent flushing and blushing. Drinking red wine produces a severe flushing of the face. There is a family history of this condition. The diagnosis is

a. Carcinoid syndrome
b. Porphyria cutanea tarda
c. Lupus vulgaris
d. Acne rosacea
e. Seborrheic dermatitis

426. A 22-year-old man from New Jersey has suddenly developed a pruritic vesicular rash on his arms, hands, and face. There are linear areas of blisters. The rash appears to be spreading for two days. Four days previously he was clearing out a wooded area in his yard. The diagnosis is

a. Chickenpox
b. Lyme disease
c. Blister beetle bites
d. Poison ivy
e. Photosensivity reaction

DERMATOLOGY

Answers

409. The answer is b. *(Stobo, 23/e, p 984.)* Isoretinoin has high potential for teratogenicity and should not be used in childbearing women unless contraception is being practiced. The drug also causes hypertriglyceridemia and drying of mucous membranes. It should be reserved for severe cystic acne. Intralesional triamcinolone is effective for occasional cystic lesions and does not cause systemic side effects. Antimicrobial therapy is of value, in part due to its suppressive effect on *Propionibacterium acnes.*

410. The answer is c. *(Fauci, 14/e, p 301.)* The rash described is classic for psoriasis. Stress and skin injury commonly exacerbate the disease. The distribution of the described rash would make contact dermatitis unlikely. Psoriasis is not contagious and is not spread by contact.

411. The answer is c. *(Stobo, 23/e, pp 651–652.)* The rash described is most consistent with Rocky Mountain spotted fever, for which a tick is the intermediate vector. Secondary syphillis could present with a macular rash in the same distribution, but the associated symptoms would be atypical. Contact dermatitis would not cause petechia.

412. The answer is c. *(Stobo, 23/e, pp 979–980.)* Contact dermatitis causes pruritic plaques or vesicles localized to an area of contact. In this case, a bracelet or wrist band would be the inciting agent. The dermatitis may have vesicles with weeping lesions. Zoster would be painful and occur in a dermatomal distribution. Herpes simplex produces grouped vesicles, but they are painful and also unlikely to occur around the wrist. Seborrheic dermatitis presents as red, scaly lesions over a circular area that appear to resolve after several hours, with new lesions developing in the nasolabial folds, scalp, and retroauricular areas.

413. The answer is a. *(Fauci, 14/e, pp 947, 1864–1866.)* Urticaria, or hives, is a common dermatologic problem characterized by pruritic, edematous papules and plaques that vary in size and come and go, often within hours. Mast cells may be stimulated by heat, cold, pressure, water, or exercise. Immunologic mechanisms can also cause mast cell degranulation. Folliculitis caused by *Pseudomonas aeruginosa* can cause a rash, often after exposure to hot tubs. The lesions would not be as diffuse, with a line of demarcation depending on the water level. These lesions are pustular, occurring 8 to 48 hours after soaking. Erythema multiforme produces target-like lesions and oral blisters often secondary to medications. Erythema chronicum migrans usually presents with a large solitary annular lesion.

414. The answer is c. *(Fauci, 14/e, pp 1864–1866.)* Avoidance of the offending agent, when it is identifiable, is most important in management. Oral antihistamines provide symptomatic relief. Agents such as aspirin or alcohol, which aggravate cutaneous vasodilation, are contraindicated. Glucocorticoids play a minimal role in management of urticaria unless the process is severe and unremitting. Epinephrine plays no role in treatment unless there is concomitant anaphylaxis.

415. The answer is c. *(Fauci, 14/e, p 1925.)* Erythema nodosum is a hypersensitivity reaction associated with this patient's sarcoidosis. Keratoses, melanoma (as described in B), and molluscum contagiosum (as described in D) are not associated with sarcoid.

416. The answer is b. *(Fauci, 14/e, pp 484–485.)* The signs and symptoms described are most consistent with scurvy (vitamin C deficiency). This syndrome can occur in older patients who are poorly nourished. Perifollicular papules develop when hairs become fragmented and buried in the follicle. Capillary fragility occurs, and bleeding into soft tissue is common. Pellagra causes a dermatitis that is symmetrical and related to photosensitivity. Beriberi does not typically cause a rash. The perifollicular nature of the bleeding does not suggest a traumatic etiology.

417. The answer is a. *(Fauci, 14/e, pp 484–485.)* Platelet ascorbic acid levels are the best approach to documenting this deficiency. Ascorbic acid, 100 mg, should be given three to five times per day until 4 g have been given. The disease is potentially fatal, and the patient should not be discharged until supplementation is guaranteed. Concomitantly, folic acid levels should be checked for folate deficiency and folate given, if necessary. Tryptophan levels are used in evaluating a patient for pellagra.

418. The answer is b. *(Freeberg, 5/e, pp 636–643.)* Erythema multiforme is often caused by drugs. It is most important to identify the offending agent. Phenytoin can induce erythema multiforme, so this information is critical. Sulfa drugs, barbiturates, and penicillin can also cause the rash. The rash, with its target lesions, should not be confused with toxic shock or measles. The sore throat is likely to be a symptom from the process itself, suggesting involvement of the oral mucosa.

419. The answer is d. *(Fauci, 14/e, pp 543–546.)* The lesion has characteristics of melanoma (pigmentation, asymmetry, irregular border), and a full-thickness excisional biopsy is required. Shave biopsy of a suspected melanoma is always contraindicated. Diagnosis is urgent; the lesion cannot be observed over time. Once the diagnosis of melanoma is made, the tumor must then be staged to determine prognosis and treatment.

420. The answer is b. *(Fauci, 14/e, p 323.)* The description and location of these lesions are suggestive of xanthoma. Eruptive xanthomas occur primarily on extensor surfaces and are associated with elevated triglycerides. Tophaceous gout can result in deposits of monosodium urate, usually in the skin around joints of the hands and feet. They may also be yellow in color. The cutaneous lesions of sarcoidosis are more red-brown in color, appearing as waxy papules, usually on the face. Treatment of hypertriglyceridemia usually results in resolution of lesions. Biopsy of xanthoma would show lipid-containing macrophages, but is usually not necessary for diagnosis.

421. The answer is d. *(Freedberg, 5/e, pp 2399–2400.)* The patient presents with the classic picture of measles. The coryza, conjunctivitis, cough, and fever characterize the measles prodrome. The pathognomonic Koplik's spots (pinpoint elevations connected by a network of minute vessels on the soft palate) usually precede onset of the rash by 24 to 48 hours and may remain for two or three days. After the prodrome of one to seven days, the discrete, red macules and papules begin behind the ears and spread to the face, trunk, and then distally over the extremities.

422. The answer is d. *(Freedberg, 5/e, pp 541–545.)* The description of this papulosquamous disease is that of a classic case of pityriasis rosea. This disease occurs in about 10% of the population. It is usually seen in young adults on the trunk and proximal extremities. There is a rare inverse form that occurs in the distal extremities and occasionally the face. Pityriasis rosea is usually asymptomatic, although some patients have an early, mild, viral prodrome (malaise and low-grade fever), and itching may be significant. Drug eruptions, fungal infections, and secondary syphilis are often confused with this disease. Fungal infections are rarely as widespread and sudden in onset; potassium hydroxide (KOH) preparation will be positive. Syphilis usually has adenopathy, oral patches, and lesions on the palms and soles (a VDRL test will be strongly positive at this stage). Psoriasis, with its thick, scaly red plaques on extensor surfaces, should not cause confusion. A rare condition called *guttate parapsoriasis* should be suspected if the rash lasts more than two months, since pityriasis rosea usually clears spontaneously in six weeks.

423. The answer is c. *(Freedberg, 5/e, pp 1482–1487.)* The patient has the typical areas of involvement of seborrheic dermatitis. This common dermatitis appears to be worse in many neurological diseases. It is also very common and severe in patients with AIDS. In general, symptoms are worse in the winter. *Pityrosporum ovale* appears to play a role in seborrheic dermatitis and dandruff, and the symptoms improve with the use of certain antifungal preparations (e.g., ketoconazole) that decrease this yeast. Mild topical steroids also produce an excellent clinical response.

424. The answer is b. *(Freedberg, 5/e, pp 36–37, 2368–2370.)* The diagnosis is tinea versicolor, which can be easily confirmed by a KOH microscopic examination. Routine fungal cultures will not grow this yeast. A Wood's light examination will often show a green fluorescence, but it may be negative if the patient has recently showered. A Tzank smear is used on vesicles to detect herpes infection. A punch biopsy would show the fungus, but is unnecessary, and the fungus might be missed unless special stains are performed.

425. The answer is d. *(Freedberg, 5/e, pp 785–787.)* Rosacea is a common problem in middle-aged, fair-skinned people. Sun damage appears to play an important role. Stress, alcohol, and heat cause flushing. Men may develop rhinophyma. Low-dose oral tetracycline, erythromycin, and metronidazole control the symptoms. Topical erythromycin and metronidazole also work well.

426. The answer is d. *(Freeberg, 5/e, pp 1609–1613.)* Poison ivy (*Rhus* dermatitis) begins 24 to 48 hours after exposure to the oil from the plant in an allergic person. Linear blisters are an important clue to the diagnosis.

General Medicine and Prevention

DIRECTIONS: Each item below contains a question or incomplete statement followed by suggested responses. Select the **one best** response to each question.

427. A 38-year-old patient presents to the emergency room with a minor injury and is found to have a blood pressure of 145/95. The best approach to follow-up of this patient's blood pressure would be

a. Full diagnostic evaluation immediately
b. Full diagnostic evaluation within one month
c. Confirm another high blood pressure reading within two months and provide advice on lifestyle modifications
d. Recheck blood pressure within one year and provide advice on lifestyle modifications
e. Recheck blood pressure in two years

428. You are evaluating a newly diagnosed middle-aged adult with diabetes. Which of the following is least likely to be of value in diabetic management?

a. Blood pressure check
b. Eye exam
c. Foot exam
d. Hemoglobin A_{1c}
e. Lipid profile
f. Liver function tests
g. Urine microalbumin level

429. In a diabetic patient, which of the following represents the currently recommended goal for blood pressure control?

a. Less than 160/90
b. Less than 145/95
c. Less than 140/90
d. Less than 130/85
e. Less than 120/70

Items 430–431

430. A 60-year-old white male just moved to town and needs to establish care for coronary artery disease. He had a heart attack last year, but gradually eliminated a couple of prescription meds (he does not recall the names) that he was on at the time of hospital discharge. However, he has been very conscientious about low-fat, low-cholesterol eating habits. Past history is negative for hypertension, diabetes, and smoking. The lipid profile you obtain shows the following:

Total cholesterol	210 mg/dL
Triglycerides	190
HDL	52
LDL (calculated)	120

To optimally treat his lipid status, you suggest the following:

a. Continue dietary efforts
b. Add an HMG-CoA reductase inhibitor (statin drug)
c. Add a fibric acid derivative such as gemfibrozil
d. Review his previous medications and resume an angiotensin converting enzyme inhibitor

431. In the preceding patient, for secondary prevention of further myocardial infarction, the patient should be placed on (in addition to aspirin)

a. Alpha-blocker therapy
b. Beta-blocker therapy
c. Calcium channel blocking therapy
d. Angiotensin II receptor antagonist therapy

Items 432–433

432. A 50-year-old white male who comes for general checkup is a healthy nonsmoker, free of hypertension, diabetes, or cardiac disease, but with a history of his 53-year-old brother having had coronary artery bypass surgery this year. You order a fasting lipid profile. Which of the following LDL target levels do you have in mind?

a. Less than 160 mg/dL
b. Less than 130 mg/dL
c. Less than or equal to 100 mg/dL
d. None specifically required based on current risks

433. In the preceding patient, if the good HDL cholesterol is found to be low, an important recommendation for trying to elevate this would be

a. Aspirin, one tablet each day
b. Dehydroepiandrosterone (DHEA)
c. Vitamin E, 400 units each day
d. Folic acid plus pyridoxine (vitamin B_6)
e. Exercise

434. A 32-year-old diabetic female who takes an estrogen-containing oral contraceptive and drinks three beers per day was found to have a triglyceride level greater than 1000 mg/dL. She is at risk for which of the following complications:

a. Acute pancreatitis
b. Sudden cardiac death
c. Acute peripheral arterial occlusion
d. Acute renal insufficiency
e. Myositis

435. A 28-year-old otherwise healthy white female on no medications presents to the ER with chest pressure, dizziness, numbness in both hands, and feeling of impending doom that began while walking in the mall. The most likely diagnosis on the differential is

a. Angina
b. Congenital heart disease
c. Gastroesophageal reflux
d. Panic disorder
e. Pulmonary embolus

436. A 45-year-old generally healthy female on no medications comes to your office with a 10-day history of nasal congestion, sore throat, dry cough, and initial low-grade fever, all of which were nearly resolved. However, over the past 24 to 48 hours she has developed a sharp chest pain, worse with deep inspiration or cough, but no dyspnea. Due to the severity of the pain, the nurse had taken the liberty of obtaining an ECG, which showed diffuse ST elevation. On physical exam you expect the most likely finding to be

a. A loud pulmonic component of S_2
b. An S_3 gallop
c. A pericardial friction rub
d. Bilateral basilar rales
e. Elevated blood pressure $> 160/100$

437. A 25-year-old Hispanic male Ph.D. candidate recently traveled to rural Mexico for one month to gain further information for his dissertation regarding socioeconomics. While there, he took ciprofloxacin for diarrhea. However, over the two to three weeks since coming home, he has continued to have occasional loose stools plus vague abdominal discomfort and bloating. There has been no rectal bleeding. The most likely cause of this traveler's diarrhea is

a. *Campylobacter jejuni*
b. Toxigenic *E. coli*
c. *Giardia lamblia*
d. *Cryptosporidium*
e. *Salmonella*
f. *Shigella*

438. A 25-year-old asymptomatic HIV-positive male comes to you for travel advice and immunizations prior to a trip to Indonesia. Which of the following would be an inappropriate recommendation?

a. Give tetanus-diphtheria booster if not up-to-date
b. Give oral polio booster if not up-to-date
c. Start hepatitis B immunization series if never received
d. Give pneumococcal vaccine if never received
e. Give second MMR if only one dose previously received
f. Malaria prophylaxis

439. In August you saw a debilitated 80-year-old female who required nursing home placement. She had had no immunizations for many years except for a pneumococcal vaccine three years ago when discharged from the hospital after a stay for pneumonia. Appropriate admission orders to the nursing home in August included

a. Flu shot
b. *Haemophilus influenzae* B immunization
c. Hepatitis B immunization series
d. Pneumococcal revaccination
e. Tetanus-diphtheria toxoid booster

440. An asymptomatic 50-year-old man who has smoked one pack of cigarettes per day for 30 years comes to you for a general checkup and wants "the works" for cancer screening. In fact, he hands you a list of tests he desires. Which test is inappropriate based on American Cancer Society guidelines?

a. Chest x-ray
b. Digital rectal exam
c. Flexible sigmoidoscopy
d. Prostate-specific antigen (PSA) blood test
e. Skin exam

441. Based on American Cancer Society guidelines for early detection of breast cancer, an asymptomatic 35-year-old female at standard risk should be advised to

a. Perform breast self-examination monthly
b. Obtain physician-performed breast examination yearly
c. Begin yearly mammograms
d. Obtain genetic testing via blood work as a baseline
e. Wait until age 40 to begin cancer screening

442. On presentation for yearly exam, a healthy non–sexually active postmenopausal 60-year-old female gives a history of having had normal yearly mammograms and normal yearly Pap smears over the past 10 years, but never an endometrial tissue sample or any screening test for ovarian cancer. The most important cancer screening evaluation on today's visit is

a. Bilateral mammograms
b. Pap smear
c. Endometrial tissue sample
d. CA-125 blood test
e. CEA level

443. You have been asked to perform a preoperative consultation on a 65-year-old patient who will be undergoing transurethral resection of the prostate for urinary retention. Of the following findings, which you detect by history, physical, and lab, which is of most concern in predicting a cardiac complication in this patient undergoing noncardiac surgery?

a. Age over 60
b. History of myocardial infarction two years ago
c. Harsh systolic crescendo-decrescendo murmur radiating to the carotids
d. ECG and subsequent cardiac monitoring showing up to 5 PVCs per minute
e. Serum creatinine 2.0 mg/dL

444. A 42-year-old Hispanic male is persuaded by his wife to come to you for general checkup. She hints of concern about alcohol use. Therefore, you ask the CAGE questions as an initial screen. These include

a. Concern expressed by family?
b. Previous Alcoholics Anonymous contact?
c. Alcohol intake greater than two drinks per 24 hours?
d. Any gastrointestinal symptoms?
e. Use of an eye-opener?
f. Presence of excess extremity shakiness?

445. A 78-year-old female comes to your office with symptoms of insomnia nearly every day, fatigue, weight loss of over 5% of body weight over the past month, loss of interest in most activities, and diminished ability to concentrate. Although further testing may be necessary, based on this history the most likely diagnosis is

a. Alzheimer's dementia
b. Anemia
c. Collagen-vascular disease with CNS involvement
d. Depression
e. Hypothyroidism
f. Parkinson's disease

446. A 65-year-old female was hospitalized for pulmonary embolus and eventually discharged on warfarin (Coumadin) with a therapeutic INR. During the next two weeks as an outpatient, she was started back on her previous ACE-inhibitor antihypertensive, given temazepam for insomnia, treated with ciprofloxin for a urinary tract infection, started on famotidine prophylaxis for peptic ulcer disease, and told to stop the over-the-counter naproxen she was taking. Follow-up INR was too high, most likely due to

a. ACE-inhibitor therapy
b. Temazepam
c. Ciprofloxin
d. Famotidine
e. Naproxen discontinuation

447. A 20-year-old college basketball player is brought to the university urgent care clinic after developing chest pain and palpitations during practice, but no dyspnea or tachypnea. There is no unusual family history of cardiac diseases, and social history is negative for alcohol or drug use. Cardiac auscultation is unremarkable and ECG just shows occasional PVCs. The next step in evaluation and/or management should be to

a. Obtain urine drug screen
b. Arrange treadmill stress test
c. Obtain Doppler ultrasound of deep veins of lower legs
d. Institute cardioselective beta-blocker therapy
e. Institute respiratory therapy for this form of exercise-induced bronchospasm

DIRECTIONS: Each group of questions below consists of lettered headings followed by a set of numbered items. For each numbered item select the **one** lettered heading with which it is most closely associated. Each lettered heading may be used once, more than once, or not at all.

Items 448–451

The initial choice of an antihypertensive agent may depend on concomitant factors. For each of the numbered conditions below, indicate the medication choice from the following list that would give the best additional benefit after blood pressure control.

a. Alpha blocker
b. Beta blocker
c. Calcium channel blocker
d. Angiotensin converting enzyme inhibitor
e. Angiotensin II receptor blocker
f. Centrally acting agent

448. Benign prostatic hypertrophy with urinary retention

449. Congestive heart failure

450. Diabetes with proteinuria

451. Migraine headache or essential tremor

Items 452–455

The choice of an antihypertensive agent may involve trying to avoid adverse effect on a comorbid condition. For each of the numbered conditions below, indicate the medication choice from the following list which needs to be *avoided* above all others.

a. Angiotensin converting enzyme inhibitor
b. Beta blocker, noncardioselective
c. Calcium channel blocker
d. Diuretic
e. Hydralazine

452. Acute gout

453. Asthma

454. Peripheral vascular disease

455. Pregnancy, second and third trimester

DIRECTIONS: Each item below contains a question or incomplete statement followed by suggested responses. Select the **one best** response to each question.

456. A 92-year-old woman with type 2 diabetes mellitus has developed cellulitis and gangrene of her left foot. She requires a lifesaving amputation, but refused to give consent for the surgery. She has been ambulatory in her nursing home but states that she would be so dependent after surgery that life would not be worth living for her. She has no living relatives; she enjoys walks and gardening. She is competent and of clear mind. You would

a. Perform emergency surgery
b. Consult a psychiatrist
c. Request permission for surgery from a friend of the patient
d. Follow patient's wishes

457. A 20-year-old complains of diarrhea, burning of the throat, difficulty swallowing over two months. On exam he has mild jaundice and transverse white striae of the fingernails. There is also evidence for peripheral neuropathy. The best diagnostic study would be

a. Liver biopsy
b. Arsenic level
c. Antinuclear antibody
d. Endoscopy

458. A young boy believes he was bitten by a spider while playing in his attic. Severe pain develops at the site of the bite after several hours. Bullae and erythema develop around the bite, and some skin necrosis becomes apparent. He is afebrile without evidence of toxicity. Which of the following is correct?

a. The boy most likely was bitten by a black widow spider
b. The boy was most likely bitten by a *Loxosceles* (brown recluse) spider
c. Antivenin is the approved method of treatment
d. The patient has necrotizing fasciitis secondary to streptococcal infection

459. A 70-year-old male with unresectable carcinoma of the lung metastatic to liver and bone has developed progressive weight loss, anorexia, and shortness of breath. The patient has executed a valid living will that prohibits the use of feeding tube in the setting of terminal illness. The patient becomes lethargic and stops eating altogether. The patient's wife of 30 years insists on enteral feeding for her husband. Since he has become unable to take in adequate nutrition, you would

a. Respect the wife's wishes as a reliable surrogate decision maker
b. Resist the placement of a feeding tube in accordance with the living will
c. Call a family conference to get broad input from others
d. Place a feeding tube until such time as the matter can be discussed with the patient.

460. After being stung by a yellow jacket, a 14-year-old develops sudden onset of hoarseness and shortness of breath. An urticarial rash is noted. The most important first step in treatment is

a. Antihistamine
b. Epinephrine
c. Venom immunotherapy
d. Corticosteroids
e. Removal of stinger

461. For which of the following categories would HIV screening be inappropriate?

a. Persons who have sexually transmitted diseases
b. Patients with active tuberculosis
c. All couples prior to marriage
d. Persons who consider themselves at risk for HIV disease
e. Pregnant women
f. Persons found to have hepatitis C when donating blood

462. A 40-year-old male is found to have a uric acid level of 9 mg/dL on routine screening of blood chemistry. The patient has never had gouty arthritis, renal disease, or kidney stones. The patient has no evidence on history or physical exam of underlying chronic or malignant disease. Which of the following is correct?

a. The risk of urolithiasis requires the institution of prophylactic therapy
b. Asymptomatic hyperuricemia is associated with an increased risk of gouty arthritis, but benefits of prophylaxis do not outweigh risks in this patient
c. The presence or absence of lymphoproliferative disease does not affect the decision to use prophylaxis in hyperuricemia
d. Lowering serum uric acid will have a direct cardiovascular benefit to the patient in lowering coronary artery disease risk

DIRECTIONS: Each group of questions below consists of lettered headings followed by a set of numbered items. For each numbered item select the **one** lettered heading with which it is most closely associated. Each lettered heading may be used once, more than once, or not at all.

Items 463–468

For each patient, select the best course of action

a. Begin isoniazid chemoprophylaxis
b. No prophylaxis indicated
c. Begin therapy for tuberculosis using three to four drugs
d. Begin therapy for tuberculosis using a two-drug regimen
e. Repeat PPD in two weeks

463. An HIV-positive patient with 5 mm PPD

464. A 30-year-old hospital employee with 15 mm PPD; previous status unknown

465. A 70-year-old new patient at nursing home with 8 mm PPD

466. A 50-year-old patient with Hodgkin's disease; 12 mm PPD, fever, abnormal chest x-ray; one sputum smear positive for acid-fast bacillus

467. A 40-year-old with 10 mm PPD; no underlying illness; first time ever done

468. A 60-year-old woman with negative PPD one year ago; now with 12 mm PPD on annual screening

General Medicine and Prevention

Answers

427. The answer is c. *(JNC VI, p 13.)* One should neither jump to the diagnosis of hypertension too quickly nor delay follow-up too long. Most patients will require a second visit to confirm the diagnosis of essential hypertension.

428. The answer is f. *(Stein, 5/e, pp 1859–1860, 1869–1872.)* All of the listed choices are very important except for liver function tests. Annual evaluation (assuming all is normal) is recommended for blood pressure checks, eye exam, lipid profile, and urine microalbumin level; evaluation every 6 to 12 months for foot exam. Hemoglobin A_{1c} (or similar test) should be obtained every six months if stable, quarterly if treatment changes or patient is not achieving goal.

429. The answer is d. *(JNC VI, p 49.)* Goals for blood pressure control and lipid levels are typically more stringent in the diabetic compared to the nondiabetic. Blood pressure less than 130/85 is recommended.

430. The answer is b. *(Fauci, 14/e, p 2146.)* The National Cholesterol Education Program includes lowering the LDL cholesterol to less than 100 in those with known coronary heart disease (secondary prevention). If dietary efforts are in place, a statin drug will likely be required. Gemfibrozil is used primarily for hypertriglyceridemia. ACE inhibitors have no significant effect on lipids.

431. The answer is b. *(Fauci, 14/e, pp 1359, 1371.)* Beta blockers are documented to lower the risk of myocardial reinfarction, whereas calcium channel blockers may increase the risk. ACE inhibitors are beneficial in this setting, but the data is insufficient regarding angiotensin II receptor antagonists.

432. The answer is b. *(Fauci, 14/e, pp 2145–2146.)* The National Cholesterol Education Program primary prevention guidelines include lowering the LDL to less than 160 if the patient is free of coronary heart disease and with fewer than two additional risk factors; they recommend less than 130 if free of coronary heart disease and with two or more risk factors. In this example, although the patient is healthy, he has two risk factors by virtue of being male age 45 years or older, plus family history of early coronary heart disease (male parent or sibling younger than 55 or female younger than 65).

433. The answer is e. *(Alexander, 9/e, p 1559.)* Only exercise in this group of choices has been shown to raise HDL. The cardiovascular system may benefit from aspirin via antiplatelet effects, vitamin E via antioxidative action on LDL, and folic acid/pyridoxine via lowering high homocysteine levels, but none of these raise HDL. DHEA lowers HDL.

434. The answer is a. *(Fauci, 14/e, pp 2142–2145.)* Hypertriglyceridemia, which is enhanced by poorly controlled diabetes, estrogen, and alcohol, predisposes to pancreatitis.

435. The answer is d. *(Fauci, 14/e, p 2486.)* Although other possibilities need to be considered and possibly evaluated, the patient's age and symptoms are consistent with panic disorder. The diagnostic criteria for panic attack are a discrete period of intense fear or discomfort, in which four or more of the following symptoms develop abruptly and reach a peak within 10 minutes: palpitations, pounding heart, or accelerated heart rate; sweating; trembling or shaking; sensations of shortness of breath or smothering; feeling of choking; chest pain or discomfort; nausea or abdominal distress; feeling dizzy, unsteady, lightheaded, or faint; derealization or depersonalization; fear of losing control or going crazy; fear of dying; paresthesias; chills or hot flushes.

436. The answer is c. *(Fauci, 14/e, pp 1334–1337.)* This history and ECG suggest acute postviral pericarditis, in which the most likely confirmatory physical finding of those listed would be the pericardial friction rub. This may be transitory and may best be heard in expiration with patient upright or leaning forward.

437. The answer is c. *(Fauci, 14/e, pp 772, 1202–1203.)* The bacterial pathogens listed usually cause acute diarrhea, sometimes bloody. They usually respond to fluoroquinolones, although some resistance is emerging, particularly with regard to *Campylobacter. Giardia* gives a more subacute-to-chronic picture as described in this patient. It responds to metronidazole therapy. *Cryptosporidium* is less common and occurs in immunocompromised patients.

438. The answer is b. *(Fauci, 14/e, pp 765–767.)* The usual immunizations may be given to an HIV-infected person, preferably as early in the course as possible, except for oral polio vaccine. OPV yields an unacceptably high risk of live virus proliferation and paralytic polio. Household contacts of immunocompromised persons should receive enhanced inactivated poliovirus vaccine (IPV-e), not OPV.

439. The answer is e. *(Fauci, 14/e, pp 762–765.)* A dT should be given every 10 years, the flu shot each fall in this age group, and the pneumococcal vaccine again at least 5 years after the original.

440. The answer is a. *(Dale, pp 8–9.)* Neither the chest x-ray nor any other test has proven to be an effective screen for lung cancer. The digital rectal exam aids in screening for rectal and prostate cancer. Other options regarding colorectal cancer are flexible sigmoidoscopy every 5 years, colonoscopy every 10 years, or double-contrast barium enema every 5 to 10 years. PSA levels, though somewhat controversial, play a role in prostate cancer screening. The physical exam remains important (e.g., in detection of testicular and skin cancers).

441. The answer is a. *(Dale, p 8.)* For early detection of breast cancer, the American Cancer Society recommends breast self-examination monthly starting age 20; breast physical examination every three years from ages 20 to 40, then yearly; and mammography every year beginning age 40. Other organizations advise mammography every one to two years from ages 40 to 50, then yearly.

442. The answer is a. *(Dale, pp 5–9.)* Breast cancer is the most common of these women's cancers. Mammography is still recommended yearly from age 50 upward (and every one to two years from ages 40 to 50, depending on the organization). Pap smears to screen for cervical cancer may be performed yearly, but after three consecutive normal exams this may be done less frequently. Endometrial tissue samples for uterine cancer become important at menopause if at high risk. There is no true screening test for ovarian cancer at present.

443. The answer is c. *(Stein, 5/e, pp 2257–2260.)* Many indices have been used to measure cardiac risk in the setting of noncardiac surgery, the most well known being the Goldman index. More recent guidelines from the American Heart Association and American College of Cardiology are fairly similar and emphasize the high-risk profile as recent MI (less than 30 days), unstable or advanced angina, severe valvular heart disease, significant arrhythmias (high-grade AV block, symptomatic ventricular arrhythmia, supraventricular arrhythmia with uncontrolled rate), and decompensated CHF. In this case the murmur of aortic stenosis is of concern. Moderate risk factors include stable angina, known *coronary artery disease,* compensated CHF, and diabetes mellitus. Low but not negligible risk factors include age greater than 75, rhythm not sinus, more than 5 PVCs/minute, evidence of atherosclerosis, and abnormal ECG, such as LVH, LBBB, or ST abnormalities.

444. The answer is e. *(Fauci, 14/e, p 2506.)* The CAGE screening tool for alcoholism consists of asking about alcohol-related trouble: *c*utting down, being *a*nnoyed by criticisms, guilt, and use of an *e*ye-opener (i.e., alcohol consumption upon arising).

445. The answer is d. *(Fauci, 14/e, p 2493.)* Depression is commonly encountered in the outpatient setting. Among the criteria for diagnosis are the presence during the same two-week period of five or more of nine specific symptoms. Five of these are mentioned in the question; the other four are depressed mood, psychomotor agitation or retardation, feelings of worthlessness, and recurrent thoughts of death (or suicidal ideation).

446. The answer is c. *(PDR, 54/e, pp 971–972.)* Many medications can potentiate Coumadin, including ciprofloxin in the fluoroquinolone antibiotic group. The other choices do not. Nonsteroidal anti-inflammatory drugs may occasionally enhance Coumadin's effect, so discontinuing naproxen, if anything, should lower the INR.

447. The answer is a. *(Fauci, 14/e, p 2513.)* The question of cocaine use must be raised in virtually all young adults with cardiovascular symptoms, despite a professed negative history. Therefore, a urine drug screen should be obtained early on. If this is negative, the patient might well need further cardiac evaluation, such as echocardiogram, ambulatory cardiac monitoring, and/or stress test.

448–451. The answers are 448-a, 449-d, 450-d, 451-b. *(JNC VI, p 30.)* Alpha blockers improve urinary outflow (and also lower cholesterol slightly). ACE inhibitors are helpful in CHF, give renal protective effect in diabetics with proteinuria, and may be protective post-MI. Beta blockers are indicated post-MI and may help tremor as well as prevent migraines.

452–455. The answers are 452-d, 453-b, 454-b, and 455-a. *(JNC VI, pp 30, 43–44.)* Diuretics predispose to hyperuricemia and therefore gout; they can exacerbate hyperglycemia and must be used with caution in diabetics. Nonselective beta blockers are contraindicated in asthma and may adversely affect peripheral vascular disease, congestive heart failure, and diabetes. ACE inhibitors are contraindicated in second and third trimesters of pregnancy due to the potential for fetal anomalies and death.

456. The answer is d. *(Fauci, 14/e, pp 6–7.)* The principle of autonomy is an overriding issue in this patient, who is competent to make her own decisions about surgery. Consulting a psychiatrist would be inappropriate unless there is some reason to believe the patient is not competent. No such concern is present in this description of the patient. Since the patient is competent, no friend or relative can give permission for the procedure.

457. The answer is b. *(Fauci, 14/e, pp 2567–2568.)* Although there is no clue to exposure (insecticides, rodenticide, wood preservatives), the clinical picture is characteristic of arsenic poisoning. Manifestations of toxicity are varied but include irritation of the GI tract, resulting in the symptoms described. Arsenic combines with the globin chain of hemoglobin to produce hemolysis. The white transverse lines of the fingernails, called *Aldrich-Mees lines*, are a manifestation of chronic arsenic poisoning.

458. The answer is b. *(Fauci, 14/e, p 2551.)* Bites due to *Loxosceles* spiders (including the brown recluse) may cause necrosis of tissue at the site of the bite. The cause of the local reaction is not well understood but is thought to involve complement-mediated tissue damage. Dapsone, steroids, and antivenin have all been used in treatment, but no therapy is of proven value. The black widow spider causes neurologic signs and abdominal pain but does not result in soft-tissue damage. Without fever and toxicity, the skin signs described are not likely to be secondary to bacterial infection.

459. The answer is b. *(Fauci, 14/e, p 7.)* The patient's autonomy as directed by the living will must be respected. This autonomy is not transferred to a surrogate decision maker, even one who is very credible. A family conference in this case would not change the overriding issue—that a valid living will is in effect.

460. The answer is b. *(Fauci, 14/e, pp 2552–2553.)* The administration of epinephrine is the best treatment in the acute setting. Epinephrine provides both alpha- and beta-adrenergic effects. Antihistamines and corticosteroids are frequently given as well, although they have little immediate effect. The patient should be offered venom immunotherapy after recovery from the systemic reaction. Removal without compression of an insect stinger is worthwhile, but not the primary concern.

461. The answer is c. *(Fauci, 14/e, p 811.)* Couples without risk factors are not necessarily recommended for HIV testing. In many areas of the country, such routine testing would result in many false-positive tests and relatively few true-positives. All patients with active tuberculosis should be tested for HIV disease, as tuberculosis is epidemic in this group. Patients with sexually transmitted disease are a high risk group for HIV disease and should be tested routinely. Pregnant women are encouraged to undergo testing. Patients who consider themselves at risk should be taken seriously and tested as well.

462. The answer is b. *(Fauci, 14/e, p 2163.)* Asymptomatic hyperuricemia does increase the risk of acute gouty arthritis. However, the cost of lifelong prophylaxis in this patient would be high, and the prevalence of adverse drug reaction would be between 10 and 25%. This expense is generally considered high compared to a more conservative approach of treating an attack when it does occur. Prophylactic therapy would be reserved for patients who already had one or more acute attacks. Although hyperuricemia is associated with arteriosclerotic disease, the association is not felt to be causal, and there is no proven cardiovascular benefit to reducing the uric acid level. In patients with lymphoproliferative disease, prophylaxis for the prevention of renal impairment is recommended. The risk of urolithiasis is sufficiently low that prophylaxis is not necessary until the development of a stone.

463–468. The answers are 463-a, 464-a, 465-e, 466-c, 467-b, 468-a. *(Fauci, 14/e, pp 1010–1013.)* Recommendations for isoniazid prophylaxis include the following (based on tuberculin reaction):

HIV-infected person, 5 mm or greater (duration of therapy, 12 months)
Close contacts of tuberculosis patients, 5 mm or greater (treat for 6 months; for child, 9 months)
Persons with fibrotic lesions on CXR, 5 mm or greater (treat for 12 months)
Recently infected persons, 10 mm or greater (treat for 6 months)
Persons with high-risk medical conditions, 10 mm or greater (treat for 6 to 12 months) [includes diabetes mellitus, those on steroids or other immunosuppressive therapy, some hematologic and reticuloendothelial diseases, injectable drug use (HIV-negative), end-stage renal disease, rapid weight loss]
High-risk group (<35 years old), 10 mm or greater (treat for 6 months) [includes those from high-prevalence countries, those in medically underserved low-income populations, residents of long-term-care facilities]
Low-risk group (<35 years old), 15 mm or greater (treat for 6 months)

By these criteria, the HIV-infected person, the 30-year-old hospital employee (low-risk or perhaps even high-risk in this example), and the 60-year-old recent converter are all candidates for isoniazid prophylaxis. The risk of developing active TB in the HIV-infected group is 5 to 10% per year and in other recent converters about 3% within the year. INH prophylaxis is most likely to be effective when infection (conversion) is recent. Consideration should be given to giving prophylaxis to all those under age 35 with positive PPDs, since the incidence of INH hepatitis in this group is low. The 40-year-old male with a positive PPD does not fall into any category of INH prophylaxis; if he is asymptomatic, no further workup would be necessary.

In contrast, the new nursing home patient should get a second PPD placed in two weeks. About 15% of these patients will have a false-negative PPD on the first test, but a true-positive on the second. The 50-year-old Hodgkin's disease patient has active tuberculosis and must be treated with a three- or four-drug regimen. The two-drug regimen is inadequate in light of emerging resistance.

ALLERGY AND IMMUNOLOGY

DIRECTIONS: Each item below contains a question or incomplete statement followed by suggested responses. Select the **one best** response to each question.

469. An important clinical difference between urticaria and angioedema is

a. Lesions produced have margins that are sharper in angioedema
b. Erythema is more pronounced in angioedema
c. Angioedema involves the deeper layers of the skin
d. Urticaria is more likely to produce symptoms of burning

470. A 20-year-old female developed urticaria that lasted for six weeks and then resolved spontaneously. She gave no history of weight loss, fever, rash, or tremulousness. Physical exam has shown no abnormalities. The most likely cause of the urticaria is

a. Connective tissue disease
b. Hyperthyroidism
c. Chronic infection
d. Not likely to be determined

471. Which of the following best describes the patient with common variable immunodeficiency?

a. The patient develops symptoms well before the third decade of life
b. At least one parent is also afflicted with the disease
c. The patient develops recurrent bronchitis and chronic idiopathic diarrhea
d. The patient should receive the standard vaccine protocol

472. A 25-year-old female complains of watery rhinorrhea and pruritus of the eyes and nose that occurs around the same season each year. Symptoms are not exacerbated by weather changes, emotion, or irritants. She is on no medications and is not pregnant. Which of the following statements is correct?

a. In this patient, symptoms are being produced by an IgE antibody against a specific allergen
b. The patient has vasomotor rhinitis
c. The patient's nasal turbinates are likely to be very red
d. Avoidance measures alone are almost always effective

473. A 20-year-old nursing student complains of asthma while on her surgical rotation. She has developed dermatitis of her hands. Symptoms are worsened when in the operating room.

Which of the following is correct?

a. This is an allergic reaction that is always benign
b. The patient should be evaluated for latex allergy by skin testing or demonstration of specific IgE antibody
c. This syndrome is less common now than 10 years ago
d. Oral corticosteroid is indicated

Items 474–475

474. A 30-year-old male develops skin rash, pruritus, and mild wheezing about 20 minutes after an intravenous pyelogram, performed for the evaluation of renal stone symptoms. The best approach to diagnosis of this patient includes:

a. 24-hour urinary histamine measurement
b. Measure immunoglobulin E to radiocontrast media
c. Diagnose radiocontrast media sensitivity by history
d. Recommend intradermal skin testing

475. Appropriate acute management for this patient would include

a. Subcutaneous epinephrine for mild to moderate bronchospasm
b. Intravenous fluids
c. Prophylactic atropine
d. Diazepam to prevent seizures

DIRECTIONS: Each group of questions below consists of lettered headings followed by a set of numbered items. For each numbered item select the **one** lettered heading with which it is most closely associated. Each lettered heading may be used once, more than once, or not at all.

Items 476–478

Match the clinical description with the disease process.

a. Wiskott-Aldrich syndrome
b. Ataxia telangiectasia
c. DiGeorge syndrome
d. Immunoglobulin A deficiency
e. Severe combined immunodeficiency
f. C1 inhibitor deficiency
g. Decay-accelerating factor deficiency

476. Recurrent episodes of nonpruritic, nonerythematous angioedema

477. Episodes of intravascular hemolytic anemia

478. Lymphoreticular neoplasm develops in patient with episodes of eczema, thrombocytopenia, and recurrent infections

DIRECTIONS: Each item below contains a question or incomplete statement followed by suggested responses. Select the **one best** response to each question.

479. Immunological mechanisms play a role in many hematological disorders. Which of the following statements is correct?

a. Warm autoimmune hemolytic anemia is less common than cold autoimmune hemolytic anemia
b. In warm autoimmune hemolytic anemia, erythrocytes are coated with IgG
c. In cold autoimmune hemolytic anemia, erythrocytes are coated with IgG
d. Complement is involved in the warm, but not in the cold, form of autoimmune hemolytic anemia
e. Corticosteroids are the primary therapy for the cold, but not the warm, form of autoimmune hemolytic anemia

480. Selective IgA deficiency is the most common of all immunodeficiency states. Study of patients who have this problem has revealed that

a. They may suffer anaphylactic reactions following the administration of serum products
b. Clinical improvement follows regular infusions of fresh plasma
c. The secretory component is usually increased in an attempt to compensate for lack of secretory IgA
d. There is an increase in 19S IgM in the secretions of certain affected patients
e. Few of them have associated autoimmune disorders

481. Which of the following statements about the administration and use of intravenous gamma globulin is correct?

a. The administration of high doses may produce a remission in idiopathic thrombocytopenic purpura
b. It must be administered slowly, as concentrated gamma globulin used intravenously has spontaneous anticomplementary activity
c. Intravenous gamma globulin preparations are safe and effective in the management of patients with selective IgA deficiency
d. In calculating the dose of intravenous gamma globulin to be administered, the physician should take into account the fact that the half-life of the immunoglobulin in the product is 7 to 12 days in vivo

482. During the primary immune response, a network of interactions is required for the successful elimination of antigen. During this process, which of the following occurs?

a. CD8-positive T lymphocytes stimulate macrophages to release interleukin-2
b. CD4-positive T lymphocytes stimulate macrophages to release interleukin-1
c. Blymphocytes react with antigen and interleukin-1 and then secrete immunoglobulin M (IgM)
d. Antigen-presenting macrophages present antigen to lymphocyte-activating macrophages

483. A 55-year-old farmer develops recurrent cough, dyspnea, fever, and myalgia several hours after entering his barn. Which of the following statements is true?

a. Testing of pulmonary function several hours after an exposure will most likely reveal an obstructive pattern
b. Immediate-type IgE hypersensitivity is involved in the pathogenesis of his illness
c. The etiological agents may well be thermophilic actinomycete antigens
d. Demonstrating precipitable antibodies to the offending antigen confirms the diagnosis of hypersensitivity pneumonitis

484. Which of the following statements concerning allergic reactions in patients receiving penicillin is true?

a. Allergic reactions occur in approximately 20% of patients receiving penicillin
b. Approximately 25% of patients allergic to penicillin will also experience allergic reactions to cephalosporins
c. Low titers of IgM antibodies specific for the "major" antigenic determinant can be detected in almost every person who has received penicillin
d. Immediate allergic reactions to penicillin, including anaphylaxis, are most commonly due to the presence of IgE specific for the "major" determinant
e. The oral route of administration of penicillin is the most likely to induce anaphylaxis

485. Immediate hypersensitivity or allergic reactions can occur in response to a variety of substances, including foods. Which of the following statements about allergic reactions to foods is true?

a. At least 30% of the adult population is believed to be allergic to some food substance
b. Breast feeding and delaying the introduction of solid foods have no effect on the likelihood that an infant will develop food allergies
c. The foods most likely to cause allergic reactions include egg, milk, seafood, nuts, and soybeans
d. The organ systems most frequently involved in allergic reactions to foods in adults are the respiratory and cardiovascular systems
e. Immunotherapy is a proven therapy for food allergies

486. A 32-year-old woman experiences a severe anaphylactic reaction following a sting from a hornet. Which of the following statements is correct?

a. She would not have a similar reaction to a sting from a yellow jacket
b. She would have a prior history of an adverse reaction to an insect sting
c. Adults are unlikely to die as a result of an insect sting compared to a child with the same history
d. She should be skin-tested with venom antigens and, if positive, immunotherapy should be started

DIRECTIONS: Each group of questions below consists of lettered headings followed by a set of numbered items. For each numbered item select the **one** lettered heading with which it is most closely associated. Each lettered heading may be used once, more than once, or not at all.

Items 487–490

For each of the following immunological diseases, select the immune defect that is most likely to be associated with that disease.

a. Decreased immunoglobulins
b. Serum antibodies to IgA in nearly half of cases
c. Decreased antibodies to Epstein-Barr virus (EBV) nuclear antigen
d. Giant cytoplasmic lysosomes in white cells
e. Abnormal phagocytic respiratory burst

487. Selective IgA deficiency

488. Common variable hypogammaglobulinemia

489. Chronic granulomatous disease of childhood

490. X-linked lymphoproliferative disease

Items 491–495

For each of the following diseases, select the HLA antigen that is most closely associated.

a. HLA-B27
b. HLA-DR4
c. HLA-DR3
d. HLA-DR2

491. Reiter's syndrome

492. Multiple sclerosis

493. Ankylosing spondylitis

494. Rheumatoid arthritis

495. Systemic lupus erythematosus

Items 496–500

Match each of the following characteristics with the immunoglobulin type that it best describes.

a. IgG
b. IgA
c. IgM
d. IgE
e. IgD

496. Binding to high-affinity receptors on mast cells via the Fc receptor

497. The only class of immunoglobulin that crosses the placenta

498. The most efficient complement-fixing immunoglobulin

499. The predominant immunoglobulin in membrane secretions

500. The class of immunoglobulin that has four subclasses with differences in their heavy chains

ALLERGY AND IMMUNOLOGY

Answers

469. The answer is c. *(Stobo, 23/e, p 663.)* Urticaria presents as discrete, erythematous lesions with visible borders, usually pruritic. Angioedema involves deeper layers of the skin. Angioedema is more likely to present as a burning sensation, not as pruritius.

470. The answer is d. *(Stobo, 23/e, pp 664–665.)* In 90% of patients with urticaria, a cause is never found. The other 10% do have underlying illnesses such as chronic infection, myeloproliferative disease, collagen vascular disease, or hyperthyroidism. There is no evidence for underlying disease in this patient.

471. The answer is c. *(Stobo, 23/e, pp 677–678.)* The patient with common variable immunodeficiency syndrome commonly develops recurrent or chronic infections of the respiratory or gastrointestinal tract. Patients have hypogammaglobulinemia, often with associated T-cell abnormalities. Diarrhea can be idiopathic, with malabsorption, or secondary to chronic infection such as giardiasis. There is no typical genetic predisposition, although clusters in families do occur. Symptoms generally do not occur until the second or third decade of life, but also may first present in the older patient. Patients with common variable immunodeficiency syndrome should not receive live vaccines such as mumps, rubella, or oral polio.

472. The answer is a. *(Hurst, 4/e, pp 172–173.)* Allergic rhinitis is caused by allergens that trigger a local hypersensitivity reaction. Specific IgE antibodies are produced and attach to circulating mast cells or basophils. Mast cell degranulation leads to a cascade of inflammatory mediators. Vasomotor rhinitis, the second most common cause of rhinitis after allergic disease, is usually perennial and is not associated with itching. In allergic rhinitis, nasal turbinates appear pale and boggy. Avoidance measures alone are often ineffective. Antihistamines and intranasal corticosteroids are usually recommended.

473. The answer is b. *(Hurst, 4/e, pp 187–189.)* Latex allergy has become an increasingly recognized problem. This is an IgE-mediated sensitivity to latex products, particularly surgical gloves. Patients present with localized urticaria at the site of contact, but can also have generalized urticaria, flushing, wheezing, laryngeal edema, and hypotension. Skin testing with latex extract confirms the diagnosis, but has caused systemic local reactions. Serum testing is definitive, but is positive in 55 to 80%. Education and avoidance of latex products is the best approach to management.

474. The answer is c. *(Hurst, 4/e, pp 192–195.)* Signs and symptoms of radiocontrast-medium sensitivity include tachycardia, wheezing, urticaria, facial edema, bradycardia, and hypotension. When these occur within 20 minutes of the injection of a radiocontrast agent, the diagnosis is made by history. No routine laboratory abnormalities are diagnostic or predicitive. Specific immunoglobulin E antibodies have not been identified, and no specific skin test is available.

475. The answer is a. *(Hurst, 4/e, pp 192–195.)* Subcutaneous epinephrine is recommended for mild to moderate bronchospasm. (For severe bronchospasm, intravenous epinephrine might be used in this patient, who does not have contraindications.) Intravenous fluids would be recommended only when hypotension is present. Atropine is given only in the setting of bradycardia. Diazepam is used when seizures occur acutely as part of the hypersensitivity reaction.

476–478. The answers are 476-f, 477-g, 478-a. *(Stein, 5/e, pp 1174–1180.)* C1 inhibitor deficiency prevents the proper regulation of activated C1. As a consequence, levels of C2 and C4, substrates of C1, are also low. Recurrent angioedema is the result of uncontrolled action of other serum proteins normally controlled by C1 inhibitor. Decay-accelerating factor is a membrane-anchored protein that inhibits complement activation of host tissue. Its deficiency predisposes to erythrocyte lysis that results in paroxysmal nocturnal hemoglobinuria. Wiskott-Aldrich syndrome is an X-linked recessive disorder associated with thrombocytopenia, eczema, and recurrent infection. There is an increased incidence of lymphoreticular neoplasm. The disease is the result of an abnormal protein present in platelets and the cytoplasm of peripheral mononuclear cells. Ataxia telangiectasia is an autosomal recessive immunodeficiency disorder that results in recurrent infection and malignancy but does not involve platelet abnormalities. It is also the result of an abnormally encoded protein.

479. The answer is b. *(Stein, 5/e, pp 661–670.)* In autoimmune hemolytic anemia, patients produce antibodies against antigens on the surfaces of their own red blood cells. These autoantibodies can be either warm-reacting, as is more common, or cold-reacting, depending on the temperature at which they are most active. In warm autoimmune hemolytic anemia, erythrocytes bind IgG, with or without complement. The IgG is specific against Rh antigens. Coating of the erythrocytes with IgG and complement leads to decreased erythrocyte survival, as these cells are phagocytized by macrophages in the spleen and liver. Corticosteroids constitute the primary therapy for warm autoimmune hemolytic anemia. Immunosuppressive drugs and splenectomy may also be necessary. Cold autoimmune hemolytic anemia may be primary or secondary and associated with such diseases as infectious mononucleosis. The cold antibody is usually IgM-specific against I/I antigens. These antibodies bind as erythrocytes move through cooler areas of the microvasculature, such as fingers and nose. Subsequently, the bound IgM activates complement, which leads to phagocytosis of the erythrocytes. Treatment consists of keeping the patient warm. In chronic cases, immunosuppressive therapy may be necessary.

480. The answer is a. *(Fauci, 14/e, p 1789.)* IgA deficiency occurs in approximately 1 out of 700 births. Failure to produce this antibody results in recurrent upper respiratory tract infections in 50% of affected patients. IgA-deficient patients frequently have autoimmune disorders, atopic problems, and malabsorption and eventually develop pulmonary disease. Replacement therapy is entirely unsatisfactory. If IgA is totally absent, its administration can represent an antigenic challenge that may result in anaphylaxis. Secretory component is normally present, and very few cases of IgA deficiency are due to a lack of this accessory factor. Some patients compensate for IgA deficiency by secreting a low-molecular-weight 7S IgM antibody.

481. The answer is a. *(Fauci, 14/e, p 1791.)* The availability of concentrated forms of gamma globulin suitable for intravenous use represents a significant advance in the management of immunodeficiency states. Immune serum globulin (ISG) could not be given intravenously, as the aggregates in the material have spontaneous anticomplementary activity and would cause an aphylactic-like reaction; intravenous preparations of gamma globulin do not have the spontaneous anticomplementary activity, but do retain the ability to activate the classic complement cascade after combining with antigen. Intravenous gamma globulin can be administered to premature babies who have low immunoglobulin levels because of poor transplacental passage of maternal IgG. Apart from its use in the management of congenital and acquired hypogammaglobulinemia, intravenous gamma globulin provides the preferable way of replacing gamma globulin in patients who are severely burned, who have hypogammaglobulinemia secondary to chronic lymphocytic leukemia or multiple myeloma, and who need IgG after plasmapheresis. Patients with selective IgA deficiency may make IgE anti-IgA antibodies that could produce an immediate hypersensitivity reaction to intravenous gamma globulin. The product is prepared from pooled plasma obtained at numerous collection sites, which ensures that antibodies to ubiquitous antigens are represented in each batch of the product. The half-life of the IgG in the product is approximately 27 days, so it can be administered on a monthly basis. Although the mechanisms are as yet unknown, it is of interest that high doses of intravenous gamma globulin (1 g/kg over five days) will produce remission in both acute and chronic idiopathic thrombocytopenic purpura in many patients. In addition, its administration has led to remission in autoimmune neutropenia.

482. The answer is b. *(Fauci, 14/e, p 1760–1761.)* The primary immune response involves an initial presentation of antigen to a CD4 inducer T cell by an antigen-presenting macrophage. The latter cell is remarkable for the strong expression of HLA-D histocompatibility molecules on its membrane. T cells, in contrast to B cells, are able to recognize antigen only in the presence of HLA molecules. The macrophage is thus able to present both foreignness (antigen) and self (HLA-D) to a CD4 inducer T cell, an essential step in initiating the immune response. T lymphocytes carrying the surface antigen CD4 (detected by monoclonal antibodies) bind to the HLA-D/antigen complex and then activate the macrophages known as lymphocyte-activating macrophages. These cells release interleukin-1, a messenger substance that binds to a receptor on the surface of the CD4-positive T cell. The CD4-positive T cell then releases interleukin-2, a second soluble messenger substance that causes the activated T cell to proliferate and produce other classes of interleukins that act on activated B cells to stimulate antibody production. Interleukin-2 also binds directly to B cells that have recognized antigen and induces them to mature into plasma cells that will secrete antibody.

483. The answer is c. *(Fauci, 14/e, pp 1426–1428.)* Hypersensitivity pneumonitis is characterized by an immunological inflammatory reaction in response to inhaling organic dusts, the most common of which are thermophilic actinomycetes, fungi, and avian proteins. In the acute form of the illness, exposure to the offending antigen is intense. Cough, dyspnea, fever, chills, and myalgia, which typically occur four to eight hours after exposure, are the presenting symptoms. In the subacute form, antigen exposure is moderate, chills and fever are usually absent, and cough, anorexia, weight loss, and dyspnea dominate the presentation. In the chronic form of hypersensitivity pneumonitis, progressive dyspnea, weight loss, and anorexia are seen; pulmonary fibrosis is a noted complication. The finding of IgG antibody to the offending antigen is universal, although it may be present in asymptomatic patients as well and is therefore not diagnostic. While peripheral T-cell, B-cell, and monocyte counts are normal, a suppressor-cell functional defect can be demonstrated in these patients. Inhalation challenge with the suspected antigen and concomitant testing of pulmonary function help to confirm the diagnosis. Therapy involves avoidance; steroids are administered in severe cases. Bronchodilators and antihistamines are not effective.

484. The answer is c. *(Patterson, 4/e, pp 479–488.)* One to three percent of patients being treated with penicillin will experience an allergic reaction to the drug. The reaction usually occurs in the first three weeks of treatment and is most common when therapy is resumed after an interruption. Allergic reactions can occur with any route of administration; however, anaphylactic or severe generalized allergic reactions are more common when penicillin is given parenterally. Penicillin reactions are of three types: (1) immediate reactions begin within 1 h of administering the drug and usually involve urticaria or anaphylaxis; (2) accelerated reactions begin 1 to

72 h after the drug is given and are manifest as urticaria or angioedema; and (3) delayed or late reactions begin more than 72 h after drug administration and typically involve skin eruptions. The degradation products of penicillin bind to serum proteins to form immunogens. Ninety-five percent of penicillin binds with protein to form the benzylpenicilloyl (BPO) group, or "major" determinant. The majority of antibodies formed in penicillin-allergic persons are specific for this determinant. About 5% of penicillin is degraded to various "minor" determinants, which include penicilloates and benzylpenicillin itself. In general, immediate reactions, including anaphylaxis, are usually due to IgE antibodies specific for the "minor" determinants. In contrast, accelerated and many late reactions are usually secondary to IgE specific to the "major" determinants. Accelerated reactions involve preformed IgE, whereas in late reactions, IgE is formed during the course of the treatment. Twenty-five percent of patients with late-reaction skin eruptions have been found to have IgM specific for the "major" determinant. Skin testing to diagnose penicillin allergy is done to both the "major" and "minor" determinants. The "major" determinant is commercially available as benzylpenicilloyl-polylysine (Pre-Pen). The "minor" determinants are tested with either benzylpenicillin G or a "minor" determinant mixture. The mixture is not commercially available. In patients with a positive history of penicillin allergy, approximately 2% will experience an allergic reaction to cephalosporins.

485. The answer is c. *(Hurst, 4/e, pp 183–185.)* The incidence of true food allergy in the general population is unknown. However, it appears to be less common than is perceived by the general population. Food allergies are considered to be more common in children than in adults. Studies have demonstrated that exclusive breast feeding can decrease the incidence of allergies to food in infants genetically predisposed to developing them. The major identified food allergens are glycoproteins. Those that most frequently cause allergic symptoms are found in eggs, cow's milk, peanuts, nuts, fish and other seafood, soybeans, and wheat. Food allergens cause symptoms most commonly expressed in the gastrointestinal tract and the skin. In addition, respiratory and, in severe reactions, cardiovascular symptoms may occur. Food allergic reactions are diagnosed by the medical history, skin tests or radioallergosorbent tests (RASTs), and elimination diets. The best test, however, remains the double-blind, placebo-controlled food challenge. If the diagnosis of a food allergy is confirmed, the only proven therapy is avoidance of the offending food. At present, there is no role for immunotherapy in the treatment of food allergy.

486. The answer is d. *(Hurst, 4/e, pp 185–187.)* The incidence of insect sting allergy is difficult to determine. Approximately 40 deaths per year occur as a result of Hymenoptera stings. Additional fatalities undoubtedly occur and are unknowingly attributed to other causes. Both atopic and nonatopic persons experience reactions to insect stings. The responses range from large local reactions with erythema and swelling at the sting site to acute anaphylaxis. The majority of fatal reactions occur in adults, with most persons having had no previous reaction to a stinging insect. Reactions can occur with the first sting and usually begin within 15 minutes. Enzymes, biogenic amines, and peptides are the allergens present in the insects' venom that provoke allergic reactions. Venoms are commercially available for testing and treatment. Within the Vespidae family, which consists of hornets, yellow jackets, and wasps, cross-sensitivity to the various insect venoms occurs. The honeybee, which belongs to the Apid family, does not show cross-reactivity with the vespids. Venom immunotherapy is indicated for patients with a history of sting anaphylaxis and positive skin tests.

487–490. The answers are 487-b, 488-a, 489-e, 490-c. *(Stein, 5/e, pp 1174–1178; Mandel 4/e, pp 1364–1377.)* IgA is present in serum as a monomer and in secretions as a polymer consisting of two basic IgA units, a J chain and a secretory component. The secretory component is synthesized by epithelial cells near mucous membranes and may function to transport IgA across the mucosa and into secretions. Selective IgA deficiency is the most common, well-defined immunodeficiency. The most common infections occur in the respiratory, gastrointestinal, and urogenital tracts. Serum antibodies to IgA are found in 44 percent of these patients.

Patients with common variable hypogammaglobulinemia are usually well until 15 to 35 years of age. They then develop pyogenic infections and have an increased incidence of autoimmune diseases. Other associated conditions include a spruelike syndrome, gastric atrophy, bronchiectasis, and pernicious anemia. Most patients with this disease have a defect in B-cell differentiation. Normal numbers of circulating immunoglobulin-bearing B cells are present, but they do not differentiate into immunoglobulin-producing plasma cells. About 10% of patients with this condition have associated T-cell abnormalities.

Chronic granulomatous disease of childhood is an X-linked disorder, with onset of symptoms during the first two years of life. Neutrophils and monocytes from these patients have a normal ability to phagocytize organisms, but have abnormal O_2-dependent killing of catalase-positive organisms (e.g., *Staphylococcus aureus, Proteus*) owing to a defect in the intracellular respiratory burst enzyme complex. Defects in both cytochrome b-245 and NADPH oxidase have been identified. Patients develop pneumonia, skin infections, draining adenopathy, osteomyelitis, and liver abscesses.

X-linked lymphoproliferative disease, or Duncan's syndrome, is characterized by a poor immune response to infection with Epstein-Barr virus (EBV). Patients with this disease are well until they develop infectious mononucleosis; two-thirds have a fatal outcome. Of those surviving the acute infection, a majority will develop hypogammaglobulinemia, B-cell lymphomas, or both. Patients have an impaired antibody response to EBV nuclear antigen. Other immune defects occur, such as decreased natural killer cell function and depressed antibody-dependent, cell-mediated cytotoxicity against EBV-infected cells.

491–495. The answers are 491-a, 492-d, 493-a, 494-b, 495-c. *(Fauci, 14/e, pp 1780–1781.)* The major histocompatibility complex is contained on the short arm of chromosome 6 and codes for three classes of cell-surface antigens. Class I antigens—HLA-A, -B, and -C—are found on virtually all nucleated cells. Class II antigens, referred to as HLA-D/DR, are expressed on B lymphocytes, activated T lymphocytes, and monocytes. Another group of antigens, belonging to class III, consists of the C2, C4, and factor B components of complement. HLA antigens play a role in immune recognition. For example, T lymphocytes recognize antigen in conjunction with HLA antigens. There is an increased risk of susceptibility to certain diseases in people who possess particular HLA antigens. For example, HLA-B27 is found in only 7% of people of Western European ancestry, yet is present in 80 to 90% of patients with ankylosing spondylitis.

496–500. The answers are 496-d, 497-a, 498-c, 499-b, 500-a. *(Fauci, 14/e, p 1769.)* Mature plasma cells produce immunoglobulins capable of combining with antigenic determinants on diverse substances. Immunoglobulins constitute approximately 20% of all plasma proteins.

They have a basic structure composed of four polypeptide chains—two light and two heavy chains. Light chains are of two types, kappa and lambda. There are five classes of heavy chains—gamma, alpha, mu, delta, and epsilon. The type of heavy chains an immunoglobulin possesses determines its class. The various classes of immunoglobulins are present in serum in different amounts and have different properties.

IgG constitutes 75% of the total serum immunoglobulins and is present as four subclasses. IgG is capable of crossing the placenta and fixing serum complement. It is the major immunoglobulin involved in secondary immune responses. IgA represents 15% of the total serum immunoglobulins and is the predominant immunoglobulin in membrane secretions. It provides primary immune protection at the mucosal level. IgM exists as a pentamerous structure and accounts for 10% of normal immunoglobulins. It plays a major role in early immune responses and efficiently activates the classic complement pathway. IgE is present in only trace amounts in serum, but is bound avidly to Fc receptors on mast cells and basophils. When cell-surface IgE is cross-linked by antigen, mediator release occurs and an immediate hypersensitivity reaction ensues. IgD represents less than 1% of normal serum immunoglobulins. Many circulating B lymphocytes have IgD on their surfaces, where its function is unclear.

BIBLIOGRAPHY

ADAMS RA, VICTOR M, ROPPER AH (eds): *Principles of Neurology,* 6/e. New York, McGraw-Hill, 1997.

AEHLERT B: *ACLS Quick Review Study Guide,* 1/e. St. Louis, Mosby-Year Book Inc, 1994.

ALEXANDER RW, SCHLANT RC, FUSTER V, et al (eds): *Hurst's The Heart,* 9/e. New York, McGraw-Hill, 1998.

CENTERS FOR DISEASE CONTROL AND PREVENTION (CDC): Probable transmission of multidrug-resistant tuberculosis in a correctional facility—California *MMWR,* 42:48–51, 1993.

CENTERS FOR DISEASE CONTROL AND PREVENTION (CDC): Update: Multistate outbreak of *Escherichia coli* 0157:H7 infections from hamburgers—western United States, 1992–1993. *MMWR* 42:258–263, 1993.

DALE DC, FEDERMAN DD, et al (eds): *Scientific American Medicine.* New York, Scientific American Inc, 1999.

FAUCI AS, BRAUNWALD E, ISSELBACHER KJ, WILSON JD, et al (eds): *Harrison's Principles of Internal Medicine,* 14/e. New York, McGraw-Hill, 1998.

FISHMAN AP: *Pulmonary Diseases and Disorders,* 3/e. New York, McGraw-Hill, 1998.

FREEDBERG IM, EISEN AZ, WOLF K (eds): *Fitzpatrick's Dermatology in General Medicine,* 5/e. New York, 1999.

GANTZ NM, BROWN RB, BERK SL, et al (eds): *Manual of Clinical Problems in Infectious Disease,* 4/e. Boston, Little, Brown & Company, 1999.

GORBACH SL, BARTLETT JG, BLACKLOW NR (eds): *Infectious Diseases,* 2/e. Philadelphia, WB Saunders, 1998.

GOROLL AH, MAY LA, MULLEY AG JR, et al (eds): *Primary Care Medicine,* 3/e. Philadelphia, JF Lippincott, 1995.

HURST JW: *Medicine for the Practicing Physician,* 4/e. Appleton and Lange, 1996.

JOINT NATIONAL COMMITTEE ON PREVENTION, DETECTION, EVALUATION, AND TREATMENT OF HIGH BLOOD PRESSURE. The Sixth Report of the Joint National Committee on Prevention, Evaluation, Detection, and Treatment of High Blood Pressure (JNC VI). Bethesda, National Institute of Health, National Heart, Lung, and Blood Institute, NIH Publication 98-4080, 1997.

MANDELL GL, DOUGLAS RG JR, BENNETT JE: *Principles and Practice of Infectious Diseases,* 4/e. New York, Churchill Livingstone, 1995.

O'ROURKE RA (ed): *Hurst's the Heart,* update 1. New York, McGraw-Hill, 1996.

PHYSICIAN'S DESK REFERENCE, 54/e. Montvale, Medical Economics Company Inc, 2000.

ROSE BD: *Clinical Physiology of Acid-Base and Electrolyte Disorders,* 4/e. New York, McGraw-Hill, 1994.

STEIN JH: *Internal Medicine,* 5/e. Boston, Little, Brown & Company, 1998.

STOBO JD, HELLMAN DB, LADENSON PW, et al: *The Principles and Practice of Medicine,* 23/e. Appleton & Lange, 1996.

ZAKIM D, BOYER TD: *Hepatology: A Textbook of Liver Disease,* 3/e. Philadelphia, WB Saunders, 1996.

Notes

- if PACs are bad – β-blocker
- Tx c̄ Warfarin 2-3 wks p̄ A-fib >48°
- Vtach is pulseless
- RArthritis rarely c̄ pericarditis but common to cause pleuritis

Notes

Notes

Notes

Notes

Notes

- Anemia of Chronic Dz
- Hep C - fatigue but not ↑ enz don't Tx
- Diverticulitis → if suspect get Xray for perf or obstx'n
  - If confirm get CT
- LBBB + ST elevation → use tPA
  - ↓T waves / ST depression
- HUS Tx → Plasmapheresis
- ITP Tx → Steroids
- vWF ↓ → cryoprecipitate
- ♀ bleeding after birth but Nl platelets / ↓ platelets → VWF / ITP
- Paget's Dz TOC (T_xOC) → Calcitonin or Bisphospho[illegible]

Notes

ISBN 0-07-135960-5
90000
9 780071 359603